THE VITAMIN D3 OPTIMAL DOSES

THE COMPLETE GUIDE TO SAFE HIGH-DOSE VITAMIN D3, MAGNESIUM AND VITAMIN K2 SUPPLEMENTATION

DR. H. MAHER

CONTENTS

DISCLAIMER

This publication contains the ideas, experience and opinions of its author. It is destined to deliver informative and helpful material on the subjects addressed in the publication. It is sold with the understanding that the authors and publishers are not engaged in providing health, medical, or any other kind of personal, professional services. If the reader requires personal psychological, medical, health or other advice or assistance, a competent professional should be consulted.

The author doesn't advocate the use of any particular healthcare protocol but believes the information in this publication should be available to the public. The publisher and author are not responsible for any adverse effect or consequence resulting from the use of the procedures, or suggestions discussed in this book.

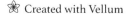 Created with Vellum

INTRODUCTION

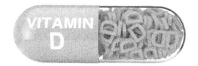

During the last two decades, no other nutrient has gained and maintained a tremendous interest in health and biomedical research, such as vitamin D.

The role of vitamin D as a hormone has gained increasing importance because of its significant contributions to good bone health and overall health outcomes. An enormous body of clinical and epidemiological studies supports today with a high degree of certainty that vitamin D is critical for the optimal functioning of most of the body's organs and systems. Vitamin D exerts beneficial effects on the brain, heart, bone, kidneys, liver, breast, lung, pancreas, thyroid, parathyroid, skin, uterus, stomach, immune system, circulatory system, muscular system, nervous system...

The idea that one can use vitamin D supplementation for a healthier, longer life is a fascinating concept. People can prevent, treat, lower the severity of many illnesses, and even reverse some chronic diseases through optimal vitamin D doses. Even more impressive is that the optimal vitamin D supplementation that promotes overall health and well-being is safe and effective.

Vitamin D optimal doses give you a safe way to improve overall health, prevent chronic inflammatory diseases, protect your vital organs, get rid of pain, aches, and fatigue, prevent cancers, and prolong life. In contrast, people with vitamin D deficiency struggle with a long list of risk factors for poor health outcomes, decreased energy, altered health, mood disorders, and more susceptibility to illnesses.

There are now several ten thousand publications that support the skeletal and non-skeletal health benefits of vitamin D. An enormous body of scientific literature currently exists. The National Library of Medicine (PUBMED database) lists ≥ 93,855 articles using the keyword **"vitamin D"** in either the title or abstract from 1928 to the present. The total includes articles that combine the use of "vitamin D" with one of the following terms:

- deficiency (≥ 35,973 publications),
- bone (≥ 28,059 publications),
- supplementation (≥ 13,740 publications),
- cancer (≥12.685 publications),
- health (≥ 8,117 publications),
- diabetes (≥7.713 publications),
- cardiovascular (≥6.556 publications),
- skin (≥5.341 publications),

- pregnancy (≥ 5,154 publications),
- liver (≥4.269 publications),
- obesity (≥4.265 publications),
- high dose (≥2.862 publications),
- brain (≥ 2.264 publications),
- vitamin D safety (≥2.251 publications),
- depression (≥ 1,485 publications)

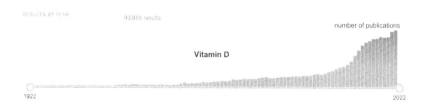

figure 1.1: increase in the number of articles published each year with the term "vitamin D" in the title or abstract (as reported in PUBMED.)

On the basis of the available evidence, optimal vitamin D3 supplementation will improve your life, help reverse some chronic diseases, and prevent many medical conditions. By taking the optimal amounts of vitamin D3—with the right amounts of magnesium and vitamin K2—, you will safely experience all the health benefits that come with it.

If you believed and followed the National Academy of Medicine (formerly IOM) recommendation of 600 IU per day in 2010, then for the past decade, you were likely vitamin D deficient. The revised recommendations by the Endocrine Society in 2011 are more realistic but also conservative, and if you got the recommended 1,500–2,000 IU per day, you were likely vitamin D insufficient. To achieve the optimal vitamin D status in the range of 40—60 nanograms/mL that will lead to lasting satisfactory status, including the winter months, you should follow a step-by-step protocol described in this book.

This book will give you ALL YOU NEED to know to reap the many health benefits of the vitamin/hormone D. Everyday patients who have decided to achieve an optimal vitamin D status by taking optimal vitamin D supplementation along with the exact amount of vitamin K2 and magnesium, continue to experience overall health improvements, less pain, increased energy, strong immune system, and reversal of some chronic illnesses such as psoriasis, asthma, multiple sclerosis. Here are some patients' testimonials:

"I'm 36 years old, female. I have been taking 30.000 IU of vitamin D3 daily for 11 months. My multiple sclerosis symptoms are all pretty much gone. My neurologist told me only to take 2000 IU a day. I did that for years, and it did nothing. Also, my psoriasis has almost all gone!" Deborah H.

"I'm 59 years old, male. In September 2020, I started taking 4,000 to 8,000 IU of D3. About six weeks later, I noticed an improvement in my general health: less pain, less fatigue, clear thinking, increased energy, and more. I had not yet started taking K2 as a separate supplement at that time, although I was already getting 100 mcg K2 daily." Michael M.

"I'm 44 years old, female. I've been taking 14.000 IU daily for the past three years, and my most recent blood test showed 55 nanograms/mL. My vitamin D levels have been varying around 43-61 nanograms/mL every six months when I get my blood test. I'm a stage 3B Breast cancer survivor, and my doctor put me on vitamin D3 supplementation. I've been in remission for the past five years. I'm in my mid 40's." Patricia L.

"I'm 70 years old, male. I was briefed that the body has trouble absorbing vitamin D3 unless one takes enough vitamin K2. After taking 10,000 IU daily of vitamin D3 and 100 mcg of vitamin K2 as MK-7, my blood pressure dropped to where I could stop my blood pressure medicines. I took carvedilol and prinzide in the morning and the evening, and now I take none. This is excellent as I was on the medicines for over 20 years!" Anthony M.

"I'm a plus-size African American, and I've been on 10.000 IU of vitamin D3 daily since the beginning of 2020. I added 100 mcg of vitamin K2 about three months ago. Not only have I not gotten even a cold, but my fibromyalgia symptoms have also dramatically subsided. I have now had the best health during these past two years than ever!" Michelle L.

"I am a professor of mathematics and was always getting colds or flu from students. I've been taking 8,000 IU vitamin D3 for about three years now, and I have not had a cold or any other disease at that time." Robert K.

About This Book

The information in this book is based on extensive research, and personal and professional experiences and represents the latest information in the fast-growing field of vitamin D and human health. I have written this book using simple language when possible so everyone can understand the content. Endnotes are included in chapters to explain some scientific terms and concepts.

PubMed database (National Library of Medicine) was used primarily for the selection of many articles used throughout this book and for the illustration of the importance of vitamin D in various fields including,

- Infections
- Cancers
- Chronic inflammatory diseases
- Pregnancy, Lactation
- Diabetes

- Osteoporosis
- Brain Health
- COVID-19
- Multiple Sclerosis (MS)
- Osteoporosis
- Rheumatoid arthritis (RA)
- Psoriatic arthritis

PART I

PART I

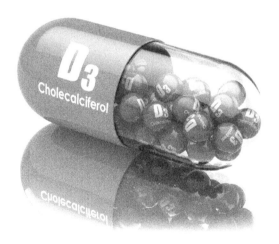

VITAMIN D - THE HORMONE OF HEALTH

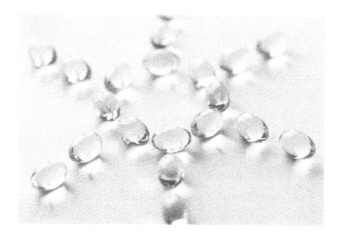

Vitamin D is known for its beneficial action in stimulating calcium and phosphorus absorption in the intestines. It exerts other valuable roles in the human body, including reducing inflammation, reducing chronic illnesses, modulating immune and neuromuscular functions, and regulating glucose metabolism.

Vitamin D's classical hormonal functions are associated with mineral metabolism and skeletal health. Vitamin D improves intestinal calcium and phosphorus absorption, promotes calcium reabsorption from bone, and stimulates mineralization of the bone matrix. The first evidence for the beneficial effect of vitamin D intake on human health came from studies on rickets in children and osteomalacia. The strategy of supplementing infants with at least 200 IU of vitamin D per day successfully reduced significantly the prevalence of rickets worldwide.

More recently, higher circulating vitamin D levels in the blood have been associated with a significant decrease in risk for a growing list of chronic diseases, including cardiovascular diseases, autoimmune diseases, bone disorders, inflammatory conditions, and various cancers. Conversely, Low vitamin D status is associated with a growing list of several risk factors for poor health outcomes, decreased energy and activity, altered health, and more susceptibility to illnesses.

A huge and growing body of scientific and clinical literature currently exists on "vitamin D and health". PUBMED (The National Library of Medicine, and the first source for biomedical literature) lists ≥ 24,401 publications using the keywords "vitamin D" and "health" in either the title or abstract from 1932 to the present, with most of the research published in the last four decades. This total includes publications that combine the utilization of vitamin D with the following terms:

- deficiency (≥ 10,529 publications),
- older adults (≥ 9,738 publications),
- status (≥ 9,088 publications),

- women (≥ 6,057 publications),
- children (≥ 5,328 publications),
- infants (≥ 2,247 publications),
- pregnant (≥ 2,180 publications),
- obese (≥ 2,102 publications),
- lactating (≥ 528 publications).

Finally, PUBMED lists ≥2,167 publications with the term *calcitriol and health* in the title or abstract, ≥5,764 articles with *vitamin D3 and health*, and ≥882 articles with *vitamin D2 and health.*

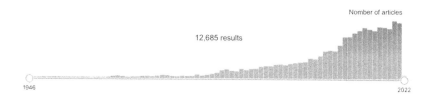

figure 3.1.1: increase in the number of articles published with the term health and vitamin D in the title or abstract (in PUBMED.)

The Hormone-Vitamin D

We always think about vitamin D as a vitamin we get from our diets, like vitamin C or B, which contributes to biological reactions that help the body operate optimally. But despite its name, vitamin D is mainly a hormone[1] and a vitamin you get on a diet to obtain a small amount of it (5—15%).

Vitamin D is characterized as a hormone because it's mainly synthesized by the human body in the skin and targets distant tissues where it produces multiple effects and contributes to numerous metabolic functions.

5

Vitamin D functions in the body like hormones do, in its myriad of effects on the body are similar to hormones' effects to some extent. Vitamin D receptor (VDR) proteins which allow the body to respond to vitamin D, are found not only in the heart, brain, lung, liver, kidneys, intestine, breast, prostate, skin, bone, cartilage, parathyroid gland but also in more than 400 tissues and cell types of the human body. Consequently, active Vitamin D, the product of the two-step hydroxylation[2] process in the liver and kidney, targets more than two thousand and a half genes producing overall health outcomes.

> The biologically active form of vitamin D also known as (calcitriol; 1,25 (OH)2D) binds to the vitamin D receptor protein (VDR). Vitamin D attached to VDR interacts with a wide variety of genes in a multitude of cells and organs to maintain cells and organ health, thereby reducing substantially the risk of chronic diseases such as cancers, cardiovascular diseases, bone disorders, liver and kidney diseases, depression.

Vitamin D - The Hormone of Health

Identified early in the 20th century, Vitamin D is not technically a vitamin but belongs to a group of fat-soluble secosteroids and is considered a prohormone[3]. The hormonally active form of vitamin D, 1-25-OH-cholecalciferol (calcitriol[4]), is converted from 25-hydroxyvitamin D3 (calcidiol[5]) in the kidneys. The classical actions of vitamin D are due to the functions of its active metabolite, calcitriol.

A growing body of scientific and clinical literature currently exists that investigates the role of vitamin D as a hormone. PUBMED (The National Library of Medicine, and the first source for biomedical literature) lists ≥ 20,727 publications that use the term *vitamin D* and hormone in either the title or abstract from 1991 to 2021. This total includes publications that combine the utilization of *vitamin D* with the following terms: hormone activity (≥ 7,980 articles), and hormone health (≥ 5,037 articles).

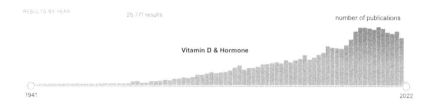

figure 3.1.1: increase in the number of articles published with the term hormone and vitamin D in the title or abstract (in PUBMED.)

The Current Understanding of Vitamin D has gone through significant changes with the discovery of vitamin D receptors in various tissues. The active vitamin D (also known as (calcitriol; 1,25-dihydroxycholecalciferol) acts in the body by entering cells and binding to the vitamin D receptor (VDR) located in the nucleus of cells. What was unexpected is to find VDR almost everywhere in the body, which implies that vitamin D can exert beneficial health effects in practically all the tissues and organs where it is located, including:

- Brain
- Bones
- Breast
- Central nervous system
- Kidneys
- Lungs
- Liver
- Endothelial cells
- Intestine
- Ovaries
- Pancreas
- Parathyroid glands
- Placenta
- Prostate

- Salivary gland
- Skin
- Stomach
- Thyroid Gland

Scientists who have mapped the points at which vitamin D interacts with our DNA[6], have identified **over two thousand and a half genes**[7]. The interaction of active vitamin D with these genes produces specific proteins with positive activities and functions. Some regulate calcium and phosphorus metabolism[8], whereas others act as sentinels of the body by preventing uncontrolled growth and then cancers, regulating insulin secretion in the pancreas, promoting serotonin[9] production in the brain, affect the immune system[10].

In other terms, vitamin D not only plays an essential role in calcium and phosphorus homeostasis but is involved in a vast range of classical and non-classical roles and functions such as cell growth[11], cell differentiation[12], and cell proliferation[13], as well as regulation of the immune system, cardiovascular system[14], nervous system[15], endocrine system[16], muscular system[17], and musculoskeletal systems.

Vitamin D also plays protective effects on many diseases like diabetes, hypertension, cancers, cardiovascular diseases, dermatological diseases, and autoimmune conditions.

The chemical structures of different forms of vitamin D were determined in the 1920s and 1930s by Windaus and colleagues'. In 1932, the biologically active form of vitamin D, found in plants and called D2 was isolated from particular mushrooms. The biologically active form of vitamin D, found in the skin and called D3, was characterized in 1936 and was suggested to result from the ultraviolet B radiation of 7-dehydrocholesterol. In 1971, studies established that the biologically active form of vitamin D and called calcitriol behaves like a hormone in the human body.

In 1980, vitamin D receptors were discovered on many cells and organs such as bone, intestine, kidney, liver, lung, heart and parathyroid gland.

In the 2010s, published studies have suggested that vitamin D interacts with our DNA, and have identified over two thousand and a half genes that directly influences to make proteins that promote optimal work of dramatically wide-ranging metabolic process, mechanism, and functions. Some regulate calcium and phosphorus metabolism, whereas others act as sentinels of the body by preventing uncontrolled growth and then cancers, regulating insulin secretion in the pancreas, promoting serotonin production in the brain, affect the immune system.

Therefore, getting an adequate amount of vitamin D through sunlight, dietary, or supplementation will improve your overall health by protecting you from conditions associated with vitamin D deficiency and possibly helping to treat them. This include:

- bone disorders[18]
- certain types of cancers such as colon, breast, ovarian, and prostate cancers.
- cardiovascular diseases.
- type 1 diabetes, type 2 diabetes, and gestational diabetes
- infections and disorders of the immune system.

- falls in the elderly.
- weight gain and obesity.
- autoimmune diseases[19].
- dementia, schizophrenia, and depression.
- multiple sclerosis[20]
- memory loss

Vitamin D for Skeletal Health

Vitamin D exerts a critical role in regulating calcium and phosphorus metabolism and sustaining healthy mineralization of bone. Calcitriol —the hormonally active form of vitamin D— elevates calcium blood levels through three different mechanisms:

- intestinal calcium absorption
- tubular calcium reabsorption in the kidneys
- calcium mobilization from the bone

1. the first mechanism is the prominent role of active vitamin D in promoting intestinal calcium absorption directly throughout the entire length of the intestine.
2. in the second mechanism, active vitamin D exerts an essential effect in mobilizing calcium from bone by promoting the normal function of parathyroid hormone (PTH) that maintains blood calcium levels and increases the number of osteoclasts, the bone breakdown cells.
3. in the third mechanism, active vitamin D and PTH stimulate the renal tubule reabsorption of calcium to ensure calcium retention by the kidney when calcium is needed.

Vitamin D

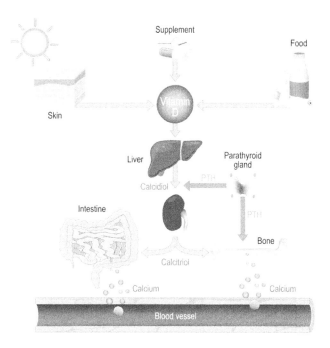

Therefore active vitamin D functions on the intestine, bone, and kidney as described above, and as illustrated in Figure 1-1, to increase serum calcium concentration.

If calcium concentrations drop too low in the blood, parathyroid hormone (PTH) will signal the bones to secrete calcium into the blood. The PTH also stimulates the production of vitamin D in the kidneys and thus indirectly improves the absorption of calcium in the intestines. At the same time, PTH signals the kidneys to secrete less calcium in the urine.

As serum calcium concentrations rise, parathyroid hormone (PTH) release decreases to keep a healthy calcium status.

When blood calcium levels become too high, PTH secretes calcitonin, which functions to maintain calcium levels in the normal range. Calcitonin reduces calcium concentrations in the blood by inhibiting the release of calcium from bones, reducing calcium absorption in the intestine, and signaling the kidneys to reabsorb less calcium, resulting in more significant amounts of calcium eliminated in the urine.

Vitamin D for Non-skeletal Health

Apart from its traditional functions related to calcium, vitamin D and its active metabolites are being increasingly identified for their overall health benefits. Emerging studies established the association between optimal levels of circulating vitamin D [25(OH)D] with decreased mortality and risk of development of several types of chronic diseases. Active vitamin D exerts many beneficial functions on the human body and promotes overall health, including:

Neuroprotective functions[21]. Vitamin D exerts neuroprotective actions involving various mechanisms. It influences neurotrophin production and release, promotes intracellular calcium homeostasis, and prevents damage to nervous tissue.

Immune system modulation[22]. Vitamin exerts a modulating effect on the immune system to prevent tissue damage resulting from an excessive response. Poor vitamin D status is linked with an increased risk of developing autoimmune diseases and infections.

Antimicrobial defense. The antimicrobial properties of vitamin D have been found effective against both Gram-positive bacteria and Gram-negative bacteria. Vitamin D has the potential to decrease the risk of infection through several mechanisms.

Anti-inflammatory actions. Vitamin D has recently been found to exert anti-inflammatory effects by regulating the production of inflammatory cytokines (cells that promotes inflammation) and inhibiting the proliferation of pro-inflammatory cells.

Anti-cancer actions. The anti-cancer property of vitamin D has been found effective and promising in certain cancers such as breast, colon, prostate, and ovarian cancers. Optimal vitamin D status is linked with a decreased risk of developing cancers and better cancer treatment outcomes by increasing cellular death in malignant cells. Recent studies linked a 4 nanograms/mL (10 nmol/L) increase in circulating vitamin D [25(OH)D] levels to a 4 percent increase in survival among cancer patients.

Oxidative stress reduction. Accumulating evidence supports that vitamin D plays a regulating role in oxidative stress and thus slows down cell and tissue damage and the aging process.

Antidepressant actions. Recent studies have found that Vitamin D promotes serotonin production and release in the brain and thus prevents depression and reduces symptoms related to depression.

Cardioprotective effects. Recent epidemiological[23] and clinical studies[24] have established that low vitamin D status is a risk factor for various cardiovascular diseases, including stroke, coronary artery disease, heart failure, and hypertension.

Cell proliferation[25]. Vitamin D exerts a beneficial effect on cellular proliferation by balancing cell growth and death. Vitamin D plays a crucial role in preventing the development of certain cancers by regulating cell proliferation and inducing malignant cell death.

Cell differentiation[26]. Vitamin D regulates cell differentiation, which corresponds to the process that enables cells to become specialized to perform a specific function. Differentiated cells are essential for overall health because they perform a specialized function in the body.

Apoptosis[27]. Vitamin D triggers and regulates apoptosis, a physiological process involving the programmed death of cells. Abnormal apoptosis is a risk factor for autoimmune disorders, neurodegenerative diseases, and many types of cancer.

Angiogenesis. Vitamin D regulates angiogenesis, which corresponds to the physiological process allowing the making of new blood vessels from the existing vasculature. Angiogenesis is required for the growth of malignant tumors and metastasis development.

---

1. **hormone** is a chemical, usually made naturally by the body, that makes an organ of the body do something.
2. **hydroxylation** refers to the process that introduces a hydroxyl group [-OH] into an organic compound
3. **prohormone** is an inactive compound transformed by specific enzymes into a biologically active hormone.
4. **calcitriol** also known as 1,25-dihydroxycholecalciferol vitamin D or [1,25(OH)2D] is the active metabolite of vitamin D formed in the kidneys that is involved in the absorption of calcium.
5. **calcidiol** is a circulating form of vitamin D in plasma. It serves as the main indicator of vitamin D status. It is also referred to as serum vitamin D [25(OH)D], and these two terms are used interchangeably in this book.
6. **deoxyribonucleic acid (DNA)**, contains the genetic instructions in humans and almost all other organisms.
7. **genes** are parts of DNA (deoxyribonucleic acid) that carries the information necessary to make a protein.
8. **metabolism** refers to the chemical processes occurring within living organisms to maintain life.
9. **serotonin** is the chemical messenger in the brain that's believed to act as a mood stabilizer.
10. **immune system** is a complex network of tissues, cells, organs, and the chemicals they make that help the body fight infections and other disorders.
11. **cell growth** refers to the increase in cell size (accumulation of mass)
12. **cell differentiation** is the process during which young, unspecialized cells take on individual characteristics and reach their specialized form and function.
13. **cell proliferation** is the process that increases the number of cells. Cell proliferation is increased in malignant tumors.
14. **cardiovascular system**, blood-vascular, or circulatory system, consists of the heart, blood, and blood vessels.
15. **nervous system** is a complex network of billions of nerves and cells that transmits signals to—and from the brain and spinal cord to—different parts of the body.
16. **endocrine system** comprises series of glands that make and secrete hormones that the human body uses for a wide range of functions.
17. **muscular system** comprises all the muscle tissues such as smooth muscle tissues, skeletal muscle tissues, and cardiac muscle tissues.
18. **Bone disorders** refer to medical conditions that damage the skeleton and make bones weak and susceptible to fractures. Some common bone diseases are osteoporosis, osteoarthritis, rickets, osteomalacia.

19. **autoimmune diseases** refer to conditions arising from an abnormal response of the immune system. Immune cells attack by mistake healthy tissues causing chronic inflammation and organs damages. Some common immune diseases include diabetes mellitus type I, rheumatoid arthritis, celiac disease, multiple sclerosis, systemic lupus erythematosus, psoriasis, inflammatory bowel disease, Crohn's disease.

20. **multiple sclerosis** (MS) is a neuroinflammatory and neurodegenerative disorder characterized by neurological deficits ranging from mild to severe.

21. **neuroprotective function** is defined as the ability for therapy, drug, or nutrient to promote and sustain the regeneration or recovery of the nervous system, its cells, neuronal structure, and function.

22. **immune system modulation**, also known as immunomodulation, is the ability of therapy, medication, or nutrient to modify the immune response, thus preventing tissue damage resulting from an excessive immune response.

23. **epidemiologic studies** refer to investigations that focus on health-related conditions and events, track their prevalence, identify their determinants or causes, determine what risk factors are associated with a specific disease or health event.

24. **clinical study** refers to research involving human participants to test how new medical therapy works in people and assess the effects and effectiveness of new medical treatments or behavioral interventions on the overall health outcomes.

25. **cell proliferation** is the process that increases the number of cells. Cell proliferation is increased in malignant tumors.

26. **cell differentiation** is the process during which young, unspecialized cells take on individual characteristics and reach their specialized form and function.

27. **apoptosis**, also called programmed cells death, refers to a mechanism that allows cells to self-eliminate when stimulated by the appropriate trigger.

2

THE MIRACULOUS MAKING OF VITAMIN D

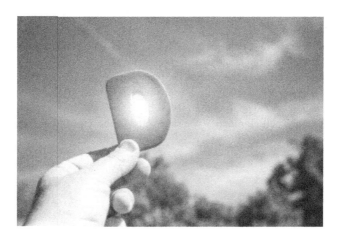

The body produces vitamin D in a chemical reaction when the sun's ultraviolet B rays hit the skin. This reaction produces vitamin D3, and the liver converts it to calcidiol. The kidneys then transform calcidiol to calcitriol, the hormonally active form in the body.

Vitamin D, first identified as a fat-soluble vitamin, is now recognized as a hormone with myriad health effects. Vitamin D is unique as a nutrient because it can be made directly in the skin from exposure to sunlight. The main forms are vitamin D2 (ergocalciferol) and vitamin D3 (cholecalciferol). Vitamin D2 is mainly synthetic (manufactured). In contrast, vitamin D3 is made endogenously in the skin from 7-dehydrocholesterol—a cholesterol derivative— and is also available in small amounts in animal-based foods or as a dietary supplement. Vitamin D2 is only available exogenously through consuming plant foods, nutritional supplements, and fortified foods. Vitamin D3 lasts twice as long in the blood as vitamin D2.

Vitamin D is used in derived terms such as vitamin D deficiency, vitamin D activity, vitamin D status, and vitamin D cofactors. Vitamin D is biologically inactive until it gets activated in the liver and the kidneys. The active form of vitamin D is commonly known as calcitriol.

For simplicity of use, the term vitamin D is generally used in the other chapters of this book to refer to both the D2 form and D3 form and their metabolites.

The miraculous vitamin D-making

Both forms of vitamin D are produced when the solar-ultraviolet B radiation interacts with a form of cholesterol. In some plants, the ultraviolet B radiation converts ergosterol —a sterol that resides on the cell membranes of fungi— into vitamin D2, also called ergocalciferol or calciferol.

In humans, when the solar-ultraviolet B radiation penetrates only the epidermal layers of skin, the 7-dehydrocholesterol into vitamin D3, or cholecalciferol.

Vitamin D3 —The Sunshine Vitamin

In 1935, 7-dehydrocholesterol—a derivative of the steroid cholesterol in the skin— was isolated by Adolf Windaus. Two years later, he isolated vitamin D3 and identified it as the natural form of vitamin D produced in the skin.

It was then admitted that vitamin D3 results from ultraviolet irradiation of 7-dehydrocholesterol. The scientific evidence behind this claim came in 1978, with more details about the stages involved in the metabolism described below.

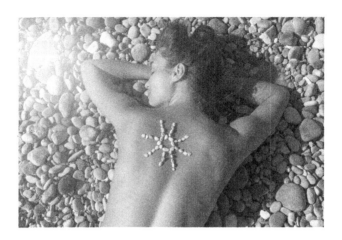

Vitamin D3 Synthesis from the skin

During exposure to sunlight, the high-energy ultraviolet (UVB) photons with energies 290–315 nanometers penetrate the epidermis, where 7-dehydrocholesterol absorbs the radiation and isomerizes into still inactive cholecalciferol, also known as previtamin D3, which is then transformed to vitamin D3. The efficiency of this conversion depends mainly on the dose of UVB, skin pigmentation and thickness, subcutaneous fat and age.

Once formed, previtamin D3 and vitamin D3 absorb solar-UVB radiation in a wide range of wavelengths. That leads, in case of prolonged exposure to solar radiation, that previtamin D3 converts to some inactive by-products, such as tachysterol or lumisterol, which have no biological effects. The quantity of previtamin D3 candidate to isomerization drops, and the amount of vitamin D3 produced is reduced consequently to avoid the harmful effect of vitamin D excess on the body.

Pre-vitamin D3 is spontaneously converted into vitamin D3 and enters the bloodstream, where it is transported by the vitamin D binding protein (VDBP).

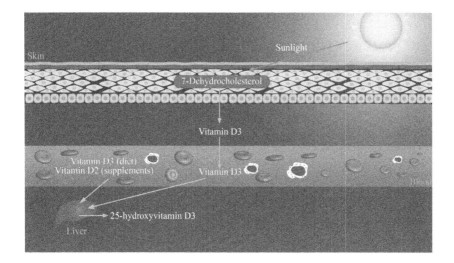

figure 1.2.1

Once linked to VDBP in the bloodstream, vitamins D3 obtained by exposure to UV-B (vitamin D3), supplements and nutrition (vitamin D3 or D2) undergo the same biological transformations to produce the hormonal form of vitamin D.

Vitamin D undergoes two-step hydroxylation mediated by specific enzymes in the liver and the kidneys. (figure 1.2.1)

- The first step in the activation of vitamin D2 and D3 takes place mainly in the liver, mediated by the enzyme called 25-hydroxylase, which converts previtamin D to calcidiol (25-hydroxy vitamin D; abbreviated [25(OH)D]).
- The second step in the activation of vitamin D2 and D3 takes place in the kidneys, mediated by the enzyme called 1-alpha hydroxylase and converts calcidiol ([25(OH)D]) to the hormonally active form, calcitriol (abbreviated [1,25(OH)2D]).

After its synthesis in the kidney, calcitriol binds to D-binding protein (DBP) to be transported in the systemic circulation to target organs.

Calcitriol exerts numerous effects in the body by entering cells and binding to the vitamin D receptor (VDR) located in the nucleus of cells. **Calcitriol activates more than two thousand and a half genes to produce beneficial health effects.**

A portion of vitamin D3 is stored in the adipose tissue for later use, which extends its total-body half-life to approximately two months in the body.

Figure I.2.1 represents all the significant phases of vitamin D metabolism:

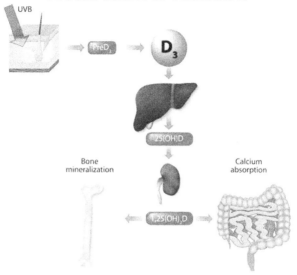

Metabolism of vitamin D

figure 1.2.2

Although the kidneys produce most of the calcitriol released in the blood, calcitriol is also made at the local nonrenal tissue by an additional 25(OH)D hydroxylation. The calcitriol made by the nonrenal tissues is not released in the blood but acts within the tissue where it is located:

- Brain
- Bone
- Breast
- central nervous system
- Lung
- Liver
- Endothelial cells (inner lining of blood vessels)
- Intestine
- ovary

- Pancreas
- Parathyroid glands
- Placenta
- Prostate
- Salivary gland
- Skin

Vitamin D vs Calcitriol: What is the difference

Vitamin D, or its two primary forms of vitamin D2 and D3, are biologically inactive and need two-step hydroxylation to produce their effect correctly in the body. Vitamin D2 and D3 are first hydroxylated in two subsequent reactions: in the liver as calcidiol [25(OH)D] and then in the kidneys to transform as the hormonally active calcitriol [1,25(OH)2D, as shown in figure 2.2.

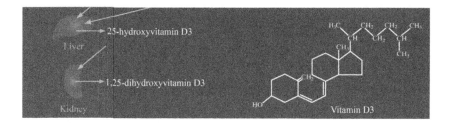

figure 1.2.3

It appears then that formally calcitriol is not vitamin D but the active form of vitamin D. The use of the term "vitamin D" to designate calcitriol is erroneous.

Implication: Vitamin D is biologically inactive before getting hydroxylated in two subsequent reactions, in the liver as 25-hydroxyvitamin D3 and then in the kidneys as calcitriol. Thus people with kidney failure could not transform vitamin d to the active form 1-25-OH-cholecalciferol (calcitriol). A supplementation of 1-25-OH-cholecalciferol is prescribed to patients with kidney failure.

For patients suffering from chronic liver disease, the trial conducted to evaluate the effect of vitamin D supplementation were inconclusive.

3

SOURCES OF VITAMIN D

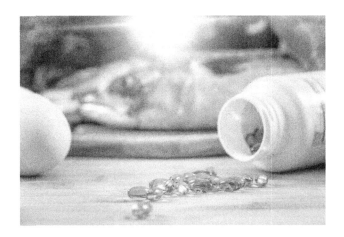

The principal source of vitamin D is through endogenous production, whereby Ultraviolet B from sunlight radiates 7-dehydrocholesterol present in the skin to form previtamin D3, which is subsequently activated in the liver and kidney. Vitamin D is also present or added to some foods and drinks and is available as a dietary supplement. Various factors and conditions affecting the skin, kidney, and gastrointestinal tract may adversely affect vitamin D metabolism.

Food and Dietary supplements

Food and dietary supplements are good sources of vitamin D, especially from October to early March (for the northern hemisphere). However, few foods naturally contain vitamin D. It's principally found in reasonable quantities in oily fish (salmon, trout, mackerel, sardines, herring, and tuna), fish liver oil, and egg yolks. Vitamin D is also present naturally in low amounts in mushrooms exposed to the sun in the form of vitamin D2.

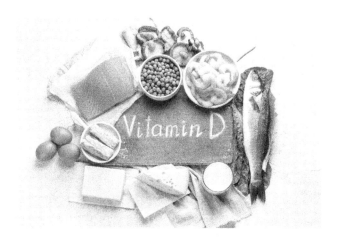

People assume by mistake that if they have a well-balanced diet, they're getting all the nutrients they need. This is not the case with vitamin D, and there is very little vitamin D from dietary sources.

> Fatty fish, fish liver oils are particularly rich vitamin D3 sources. Wild fatty fishes can provide significant amounts of vitamin D thanks to their vitamin D rich alimentation. However, farm-raised fatty fishes (salmon, trout...) contain less amounts of vitamin D unless it has been added as a supplement to their alimentation.

Many frequently consumed foods have been fortified with vitamin D in the last decades, such as milk, dairy products, and cereals. Based on data from the United States Food and Drug Administration (FDA), almost all fluid dairy, more than 50 percent of all milk substitutes, more than 80 percent of ready-to-eat breakfast cereals, more than one-quarter of yogurts, and approximately 15 percent of cheeses, spreads, and juices, are fortified with vitamin D in the USA.

In Canada, cow's milk is fortified with 2.2 to 2.9 µg (88 to 117 IU) of vitamin D3 per 250 mL. All kinds of margarine are also fortified with vitamin D 13.25 µg (530 IU) per 100 g.

However, there are less than 120 IU in a cup of milk (250 mL) or vitamin D-fortified juice. Multivitamins are poor in vitamin D; even manufacturers claim they contain 100 percent of the recommended daily allowance (RDAs). Because the published RDAs are based on outdated and erroneous USDA recommendations (for more details, please refer to the chapter "Vitamin D Requirements - The Big Mistake"). And taking several tablets won't solve the problem and may be harmful because of vitamin A toxicity.

Here is a table of the Vitamin D Content of Selected Foods:

- **Cod liver oil** : 34.0 mcg | 1,360 IU per 1 tablespoon. Be aware that just one tablespoon of cod liver oil can fulfill up to 250% of your daily vitamin A needs in one serving. **And that prolonged daily intake of vitamin A may induce severe**

toxicity with various damages, including jaundice, liver injury, enlargement of the liver, and cirrhosis.

- **Trout (rainbow), farmed, cooked:** 16.2 mcg | 645 IU per 3 ounces
- **Salmon, cooked,** 3 ounces: 14.2 mcg | 570 IU per 3 ounces

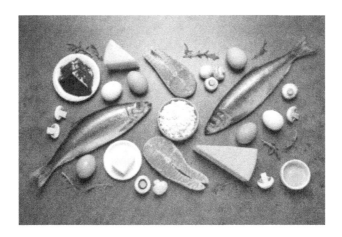

- **Swordfish (cooked).** 3 ounces: 14.15 mcg | 566 IU
- **Mushrooms, white, raw, sliced,** exposed to UV light: 9.2 mcg | 366 IU per ½ cup
- **Milk, 2% milkfat, vitamin D fortified:** 2.9 mcg | 120 IU per 1 cup
- **Milk, fortified.** 1 cup: 2.87-3.1 mcg | 115-124 IU.
- **Soy, almond, and oat milk,** vitamin D fortified, various brands: 2.5-3.6 mcg | 100-144 IU per 1 cup
- **Ready-to-eat cereal, fortified with 10% of the daily value for vitamin D:** 2.0 mcg | 80 IU per 1 serving
- **Orange juice, fortified.** 1 cup: 3.45 mcg | 137 IU.
- **Yogurt, fortified with 20% of the DV of vitamin D.** 6 ounces: 2.0 mcg | 80 IU.
- **Sardines (Atlantic), canned in oil, drained:** 1.2 mcg | 46 IU per 2 sardines
- **Egg, 1 large, scrambled:** 1.1 mcg | 44 IU per 1 egg
- **Egg yolk:** 1 large egg: 1.0 mcg | 41 IU

- Liver, beef, braised: 1.0 mcg | 40 IU per 3 ounces
- Tuna fish (light), canned in water, drained: 1.0 mcg | 40 IU per 3 ounces
- Cheese, cheddar: 0.4 mcg | 17 IU per 1.5 ounce
- Mushrooms, portabella, raw, diced: 0.1 mcg | 4 IU per ½ cup
- Swiss cheese. 1 ounce: 0.15 mcg | 6 IU.
- Chicken breast, roasted: 0.1 mcg | 4 IU per 3 ounces
- Beef, ground, 90% lean, broiled: 0.0 mcg | 1.7 IU per 3 ounces
- Broccoli, raw, chopped: 0.0 mcg | 0 IU per ½ cup
- Carrots, raw, chopped, ½ cup: 0.0 mcg | 0 IU per ½ cup
- Almonds, dry roasted: 0.0 mcg | 0 IU per 1 ounce
- Apple, large: 0.0 mcg | 0 IU
- Banana, large: 0.0 mcg | 0 IU
- Rice, brown, long-grain, cooked: 0.0 mcg | 0 IU per 1 cup
- Whole wheat bread: 0.0 mcg | 0 IU per 1 slice
- Lentils, boiled: 0.0 mcg | 0 IU per ½ cup
- Sunflower seeds, roasted: 0.0 mcg | 0 IU per ½ cup
- Edamame, shelled, cooked: 0.0 mcg | 0 IU per ½ cup
- Margarine, fortified. 1 tablespoon: 60 IU.

table 1. 3.1

The Sun

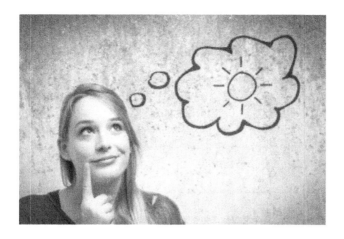

What is ultraviolet radiation?

The vitamin D production miracle starts when sun radiations hit our skin. The sun's emissions include heat, visible light, ultraviolet and other radiations. These solar irradiances are characterized by their wavelength—the longer the photon's wavelength, the lower its energy—.

Ultraviolet light falls in the range of electromagnetic radiation between visible light and x-rays (wavelength 400 to 200 nm). Ultraviolet radiation is divided into three bands:

- UVA: radiation that extends from about 320 to 400 nm in wavelength. UVA rays contain much less energy than UVB and penetrate the lower layers of the epidermis, causing skin tanning and wrinkles and contributing to the skin aging process. UVA is thought to cause skin cancer.
- UVB: radiation that extends from about 280 to 320 nm in wavelength. UVB is mainly responsible for sunburn, skin aging, and skin cancer. **UVB is the only form of solar-ultraviolet radiation that triggers vitamin D production in the skin.**
- UVC: radiation that extends from about 200 to 280 nm in

wavelength. UVC is absorbed mainly by the upper
atmosphere of the earth.

> In the case of prolonged exposure to sunlight, previtamin D3
> converts to number of inactive by-products, such as tachysterol or
> lumisterol which have no biological effects. This photoconversion
> of previtamin D3 prevent the production to toxic amounts of D3.

The vitamin-Hormone

Vitamin D is a vitamin/hormone that is produced by direct exposure
to sunlight. Vitamin D3 is then synthesized in the skin from 7-dehy-
drocholesterol —that functions in the serum as a cholesterol
precursor— as a result of direct exposure to the solar-ultraviolet B
radiation (290-320 nm). The absorbed energy by the skin causes
chemical changes within the 7-dehydrocholesterol, resulting in the
formation of previtamin D3.

In the epidermis, previtamin D3 undergoes rapid, thermally-induced
conversion to vitamin D3, as illustrated in figure 3.1.

Once formed, vitamin D3 and previtamin D3 continue to absorb UV
radiation and reach a steady state in case of prolonged exposure that
results in the breakdown of these molecules into biologically inactive
photoproducts such as tachysterol or lumisterol. For this reason,
during prolonged exposure to solar-UVB radiation, only 10–15% of 7-
dehydrocholesterol is converted to previtamin D3, preventing intoxication by high levels of vitamin D.

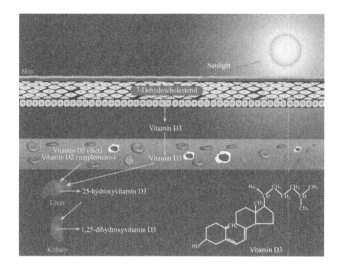

figure 1.3.1

Vitamin D3 is inactive until it undergoes two-step hydroxylation2. It is first activated in the liver to calcidiol3. The serum half-life of vitamin D metabolite [25(OH)D] is approximately 15 days. Vitamin D metabolite [25(OH)D] is activated in the kidney into the hormonal form calcitriol5.

The peak of vitamin D3 metabolite [25(OH)D] serum levels is observed 24 to 48 h after exposure to ultraviolet B radiation. Levels of vitamin D3 metabolites decline exponentially after that. Excess vitamin D3 is stored in the adipose tissue, which prolongs its half-life in the human body to roughly two months.

Factors influencing cutaneous vitamin D3 synthesis

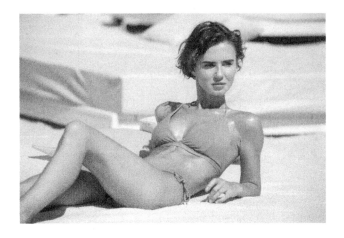

The production of vitamin D3 in human skin is a function of the amount of solar-ultraviolet B radiation reaching the dermis and the availability of 7- dehydrocholesterol. Therefore, numerous factors influence the photosynthesis efficiency and the bioavailability of vitamin D and contribute to the risk of vitamin D insufficiency or deficiency. These factors are divided into two different categories:

- factors that influence the number of ultraviolet UVB photons that strike human skin, like atmospheric components, geographic location, season, time of day, clothing, sunscreen use, and skin pigmentation.
- factors and disorders that affect the availability of 7-dehydrocholesterol such as age, obesity, and the impact of some chronic illnesses.

Geographic location

Solar zenith angle is one of the most important factors controlling UVB radiation reaching the earth's surface.

In the Northern Hemisphere, during the summer season, the radiations from the sun hit the earth's surface more directly than at any other season. Ultraviolet B radiation that hits the skin is maximal, and you can get the most sun and UVB penetration.

When the zenith angle is more oblique, the UVB radiation traverses a long path through the stratospheric ozone layer, which decreases the number of UVB radiation reaching the earth's surface. That is the explanation the skin produces little if any, vitamin D3 from the sunlight at latitudes low than 37 degrees south of the equator and above 37 degrees north when the solar rays are more oblique during the autumn and winter months.

During winter, Northern Hemisphere is tilted away from the sun, and the angle that sunlight passes through the atmosphere is more oblique.

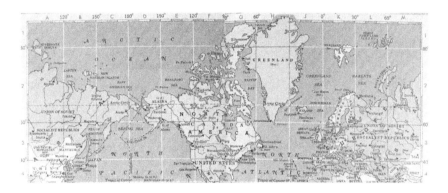

People who live above the 37-degree latitude line —roughly the imaginary line between Philadelphia and San Francisco— get little to no UVB exposure between the autumn and winter months to make vitamin D.

Type of Skin

Human skin color displays variations throughout life and is influenced by several factors such as race, age, sex and hormones. However, the most important factors that determine human skin color are the quantity of melanin8 pigment and its chemical structure. Melanin, the pigment responsible for the difference in skin color among racial groups, acts as a powerful natural sunscreen that efficiently absorbs solar-UVB photons and thus substantially diminishes the production of vitamin D3 in the skin.

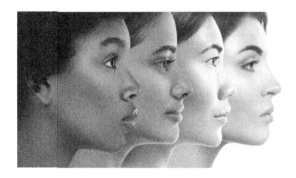

This inhibitory effect on Cutaneous Vitamin D production increases with skin color. Hence, dark-skinned people require more sunlight exposure than fair or light-skinned people to produce an equivalent vitamin D.

Sunscreens use

Sunscreens prevent sunburn, skin aging and skin cancer by blocking the UVB light. A sunscreen with a sun protection factor of 15 (SPF 15) filters 93 percent of UVB rays and thus reduces vitamin D3 biosynthesis by the same degree.

SPF 30 Sunscreens filter 97 percent of UVB photons, and SPF 50 blocks out 98 percent. That leaves only 2 to 7 percent of solar-UVB reaching human skin, consequently decreasing vitamin D3 biosynthesis.

Age

In one study, researchers conducted a large evaluation of surgically obtained skin (age range between 8 and 92 years) to identify if the cutaneous production of vitamin D3 is age-dependent. Skins were exposed to ultraviolet radiation, and the contents of previtamin D3 were determined in the epidermis and dermis.

The researchers found that aging can significantly decrease the ability of the skin to produce previtamin D3 (by greater than twofold).

Compared with younger, the elderly have lower levels of the 7-dehydrocholesterol in the skin that UVB light converts into the previtamin D3.

Obesity

Obesity is a severe health condition that may also be linked to poor cutaneous vitamin D production. Studies evaluated the production of vitamin D3 following whole-body irradiation in obese and nonobese subjects. The circulating vitamin D [25(OH)D] concentrations in participants' blood showed that the resulting increase in vitamin D3 was 57 percent lower in obese than in nonobese subjects. Similar observations occurred after an oral dose of 50,000 IU of vitamin D.

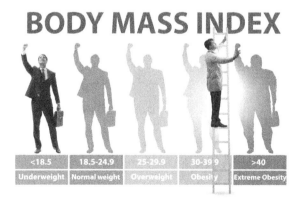

The reason for this obesity-associated vitamin D deficiency is not clear, although several studies. Some studies have suggested that the excess fat in obese patients absorbs and keeps the vitamin D trapped so that it cannot be used to properly mineralize the skeleton or maintain cellular health.

Vitamin D2 Versus Vitamin D3

Multiple dietary forms of vitamin D are commercially available for supplement use. The two most common dietary supplements are vitamin D2 (ergocalciferol), derived from non-vertebrate species (fungi, plants, and invertebrates), and vitamin D3 (cholecalciferol), derived from vertebrates.

Both forms of vitamin D are produced when the solar-ultraviolet B radiation interacts with a form of cholesterol. In some plants, the ultraviolet B radiation converts ergosterol —a sterol that resides on the cell membranes of fungi— into vitamin D2, which is also called ergocalciferol or calciferol.

In humans, when the solar-ultraviolet B radiation penetrates only the epidermal layers of skin, the 7-dehydrocholesterol into vitamin D3, or cholecalciferol.

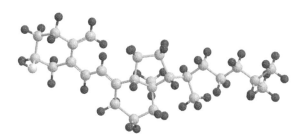

Vitamins D2 and D3 differ only slightly in their side-chain structure, and both have been extensively used to treat vitamin D deficiency rickets9 and osteomalacia10 in adults and suboptimal vitamin D status. Physiological actions of these two steroid hormones include calcium and phosphorus homeostasis, cell cycling and proliferation11, cell differentiation12, and apoptosis13.

Early studies suggested these two forms of vitamin D as equipotent and interchangeable in humans. However, recent studies showed that vitamin D2 was by far less effective than vitamin D3 in increasing serum level of 25(OH)D—the indicator of vitamin D insufficiency and deficiency in the blood—. One study in 2011 found that vitamin D3 (cholecalciferol) is 87 percent more potent than Vitamin D2 (ergocalciferol). Another study determined that the same single dose of vitamin D2 does not last longer than the dose of D3.

In other terms, in humans, vitamin D3 provides greater benefits than vitamin D2. Therefore, vitamin D3 should be considered the preferred treatment or supplementation option.

4

VITAMIN D MISCONCEPTIONS

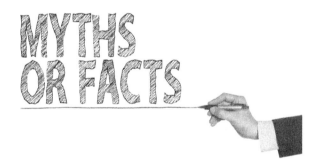

Misconceptions and myths about vitamin D continue to grow despite thousands of clinical, epidemiological, and observational studies in the last two decades.

There are many misconceptions about vitamin D. Part of these misconceptions are because vitamin D is fat-soluble and the widespread belief that fat-soluble supplements are dangerous at high doses.

1. Vitamin D Is a Vitamin

We always think about vitamin D as a vitamin we get from our diets, like vitamin C or B, which contributes to biological reactions that help the body operate optimally. But despite its name, vitamin D is mainly a hormone and a vitamin you get on a diet to obtain a small amount of it (5—15%).

Vitamin D is characterized as a hormone because it's mainly synthesized by the human body in the skin and targets distant tissues where it produces multiple effects and contributes to numerous metabolic functions.

2. Vitamin D is considered a hormone because the body synthesizes it.

Not only. Vitamin D is recognized as a hormone because it's primarily made by the human body in the skin and activated in the liver and kidneys into it hormonally form calcitriol.

Vitamin D functions in the body as hormones do, and its myriad effects on the body are similar to hormones' effects to some extent. Vitamin D receptor (VDR) proteins which allow the body to respond to vitamin D, are found not only in the heart, lung, liver, kidneys, intestine, skin, bone, cartilage, and parathyroid gland but also in more than 400 tissues and cell types of the human body. Consequently, active Vitamin D, the product of the two-step hydroxylation process in the liver and kidney, targets more than two thousand genes and is associated with overall health outcomes.

3. It's Easy to Get sufficient Vitamin D Through Diet Alone.

Few foods naturally contain vitamin D. It's principally found in reasonable quantities in oily fish (salmon, trout, mackerel, sardines, herring, and tuna), fish liver oil, and egg yolks. People assume that if they have a well-balanced diet, they're getting all the nutrients they need. That is not the case with vitamin D, and there is petite vitamin D from dietary sources. Vitamin D is also present naturally in low amounts in mushrooms exposed to the sun in the form of vitamin D2. These foods contain only a small fraction of the daily value (DV) of vitamin D.

Many frequently consumed foods have been fortified with vitamin D in the last decades, such as milk, dairy products, and cereals. However, there are less than 120 IU in a cup of milk (250 mL) or vitamin D-fortified juice.

Cod liver oil, used for centuries to prevent rickets, contains high amounts of vitamin D (450 IU per teaspoon). However, due to its high content of vitamin A, you can not rely on it for prolonged consumption. Vitamin A is known to cause severe toxicity.

So, getting sufficient vitamin D through food alone is practically impossible.

4. Everyone Should Get Their Vitamin D Blood Levels Tested.

The vitamin D blood level test may be requested for several reasons. Most experts agree that we should systematically check vitamin D levels in high-risk people. These include:

- dark-skinned people
- obese people
- people with skeletal disorders (e.g., osteoporosis, osteomalacia, osteopenia)
- people with gastrointestinal disorders (e.g., inflammatory bowel disease)
- people with anorexia nervosa
- people who had gastric bypass surgeries
- people with chronic kidney disease
- chronic liver diseases
- people with celiac disease or sprue

- people with endocrine disorders
- pregnant and lactating women

Your doctor may suspect a low vitamin D level. If this is the case taking a Vitamin D3 supplement may be sufficient.

5. Everyone Should Take the Same Amount of Vitamin D Regardless of Weight, Age, and Skin Color

The vitamin D needs of everyone are different and are affected by several factors, including residence latitude, season, time of day, clothing, age, obesity, sunscreen use, skin type, and the incidence of some chronic illnesses.

6. Vitamin D toxicity frequently occurs when an excess of vitamin D is taken (over 4,000 IU per day)

Vitamin D toxicity is rare and occurs only when a person gets very high doses (over 50,000 IU per day) for months or years. For adults, two clinical studies have established that taking 250 mcg (10.000 IU) per day of vitamin D is considered safe with no observed adverse effect level (NOAEL).

Other clinical studies assessed the safety of vitamin D3 therapy based on 50,000-100,000 IU/week. Adults with statin intolerance were given 50,000-100,000 IU/week for 12 months with no sign of toxicity. Their vitamin D [25(OH)D] level rarely exceeded 100 nanograms/mL but never reached toxic levels.

7. Vitamin D is the "bone health" hormone due to its properties in treating and preventing bone diseases

Besides playing crucial roles in calcium and phosphorus metabolism and bone mineralization, vitamin D has been recognized since the 1980s as playing a vast range of classical and non-classical roles and functions, such as cellular growth, cellular proliferation, cellular differentiation, as well as supporting immune health, brain health, nervous system health, supporting lung function, musculoskeletal and cardiovascular health.

Vitamin D also plays protective effects on many diseases like diabetes, hypertension, cancers, cardiovascular diseases, dermatological diseases, and autoimmune conditions.

8. Government Recommended Daily Intake for Are adequate

The Government Recommended Daily Intakes (RDAs) are miscalculated and erroneous. A statistical error in calculating the recommended dietary allowances (RDAs) for vitamin D was discovered first in 2014 and confirmed by another study in 2015. Using the data of the Institute of Medicine mandated by the United States and Canadian governments, investigators Veugelers and Ekwaru found that 8895 IU per day was needed for 97.5% of individuals to achieve values ≥50 nmol/L (20 nanograms/mL). Therefore, the correctly calculated RDA for vitamin D is 8895 IU per day (instead of 600 IU, the published IOM RDAs) for individuals aged 1 to 70 years.

Another study published one year later in 2015, confirmed that the Institute of Medicine had made a serious calculation error and established that the total intake required to achieve 50 nmol/L (20 nanograms/mL) in 97.5% of individuals must be close to 7000 IU per day, not substantially different from the correctly calculated RDA by Veugelers and Ekwaru.

9. Vitamin D2 and Vitamin D3 are equivalent and equal

The two most common dietary supplements are vitamin D2 (ergocalciferol), derived from non-vertebrate species (fungi, plants, and invertebrates) and vitamin D3 (cholecalciferol), derived from vertebrates.

Vitamins D2 and D3 differ only slightly in their side-chain structure. Both have been extensively used to treat vitamin D deficiency rickets and osteomalacia in adults and suboptimal vitamin D status. Physiological actions of these two steroid hormones18 include calcium and phosphorus homeostasis, cell cycling and proliferation, cell differentiation, and apoptosis.

Early studies suggested these two forms of vitamin D as equipotent and interchangeable in humans. However, recent studies showed that vitamin D2 was by far less effective than vitamin D3 in increasing serum level of 25(OH)D—the indicator of vitamin D insufficiency and deficiency in the blood—. One study in 2011 found that vitamin D3 (cholecalciferol) is 87 percent more potent than Vitamin D2 (ergocalciferol). Another study determined that the same single dose of vitamin D2 does not last longer than D3.

In other terms, in humans, vitamin D3 provides greater benefits than vitamin D2. Therefore, vitamin D3 should be considered the preferred treatment or supplementation option.

10. Excessive exposure to sunlight poses no risk of vitamin D toxicity

During prolonged sunlight exposure, when the concentration of vitamin D precursors formed in the skin reaches a certain level, relevant regulatory mechanisms in the skin function to degrade the excessive production of vitamin D3 and prevent

Cutaneous production with total body exposure to solar-ultraviolet B may be comparable in some specific conditions (latitude, skin type, age, weight status) to taking an oral dose between 250—500 mcg (10,000—20,000 IU) per day.

During the summer months, people who consume 10,000 International Units of the vitamin D3 per day, and get long daily sunbaths with total body exposure, can reach a level of 500—750 mcg (20,000—30,000 IU). In this case, they may reduce their dietary intake or sun exposure. Therefore, excessive exposure to sun rays is considered safe regarding vitamin D status.

5

MAGNESIUM, THE KEY TO VITAMIN D BENEFITS

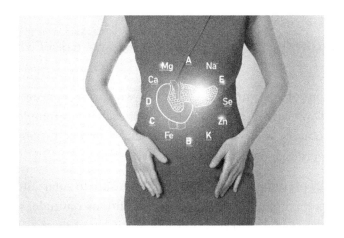

" People taking vitamin D supplements may see little to no improvement in their overall health if they have a magnesium deficiency. Poor magnesium status may expose people to vitamin D deficiency even if they get adequate sun exposure or optimal vitamin D supplementation. Because, without magnesium, Vitamin D remains stored and inactive. In contrast, People with sufficient magnesium levels require less

Vitamin D supplementation to achieve optimum Vitamin D levels considered adequate for overall health.

Nutrients usually act in a combined way in the human body. Thus, to a certain extent, intestinal absorption and subsequent metabolism of a particular nutrient depend on other nutrients' availability. These vitamins and minerals are called cofactors or "helper nutrients".

Adequate vitamin D levels require more than sun exposure, a balanced diet, and taking dietary supplements. Achieving optimal vitamin D levels in the range of 40 to 60 nanograms/ml (100 to 150 nmol/L) depends on taking the right amounts of cofactors: magnesium and vitamin K.

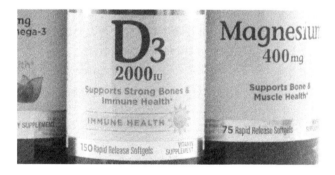

The indispensable role of Magnesium

Magnesium is an essential nutrient to the human body, playing an indispensable role in promoting and sustaining health and life. As a critical cofactor for activating a wide range of metabolic enzymes[1] and cell transporters, magnesium is involved in several hundred chemical reactions in the body and is required by every cell. It is indispensable in hormone secretion, energy metabolic processes, mineral absorption, nervous tissue conduction, protein synthesis, blood clotting, neuromuscular excitability, insulin function, and muscle contraction.

Magnesium is also indispensable to activate vitamin D because the hydroxylation[2] of vitamin D in the liver and kidneys is mediated by enzymes that require magnesium.

As noted in the chapter "Vitamin D - The Hormone of health", vitamin D is biologically inactive until it undergoes two-step hydroxylation in the liver and the kidneys. In the liver, 25-Hydroxylase synthesizes calcidiol [25(OH)D] from vitamin D3 or vitamin D2, and then 1α-hydroxylase transforms calcidiol [25(OH)D] into active calcitriol [1,25(OH)2D] in the kidney. Both 25-Hydroxylase and 1α-hydroxylase enzymes are magnesium-dependent.

Emerging scientific and clinical literature currently exists for vitamin D and Magnesium due to the increasing awareness concerning the role of cofactors in vitamin D adequacy. PUBMED (The National Library of Medicine, and the first source for biomedical literature) lists ≥ 2,401 publications that use the keywords **"vitamin D"** and **"magnesium"** in either the title or abstract from 1946 to the present, with most of the research published in the last two decades. This total includes publications that combine one of the following terms with vitamin D:

- magnesium *deficiency* (≥ 684 articles),
- magnesium status (≥ 474 articles),
- magnesium activation (≥469 articles),
- magnesium role (≥ 374 articles),
- magnesium supplementation (≥369 articles).

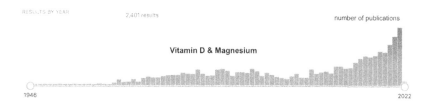

figure 3.1.1: increase in the number of articles published with the term magnesium and vitamin D in the title or abstract (in PUBMED.)

Poor magnesium status may expose people to vitamin D deficiency even if they get adequate sun exposure or optimal vitamin D supplementation.

Therefore, without a sufficient amount of magnesium, only the activated fraction could affect the human body. The remaining vitamin D will stay inactive and unable to deliver the expected health outcomes. In turn, taking high doses of vitamin D can induce severe magnesium depletion.

To address this problem, when increasing your circulating vitamin D [25(OH)D] to the optimal range of 40-60 nanograms/mL (overall health range) or 50-80 nanograms/mL (preventive cancer range), you should take an adequate magnesium supplementation for optimal results and outcomes.

People taking vitamin D supplements may see little to no improvement in their overall health if they have a magnesium deficiency. Because, without enough magnesium, Vitamin D remains stored and inactive. In contrast, People with high magnesium levels require less Vitamin D supplementation to achieve optimum Vitamin D levels considered adequate for overall health.

Magnesium Deficiency

Like vitamin D, magnesium is used by practically all the organs in the human body, and its deficiency may lead to several chronic illnesses.

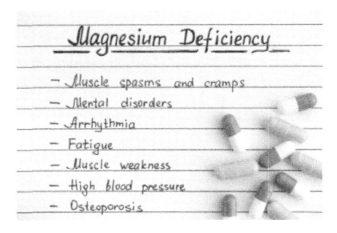

Magnesium Deficiency

- Muscle spasms and cramps
- Mental disorders
- Arrhythmia
- Fatigue
- Muscle weakness
- High blood pressure
- Osteoporosis

The 2015 Dietary Guidelines Advisory Committee (DGAC) determined that vitamin A, vitamin D, vitamin E, calcium, and magnesium are under-consumed relative to the Estimated Average Requirement (EAR) in the U.S. population. The DGAC also determined that vitamin A, vitamin D, vitamin E, magnesium, and calcium were shortfall nutrients.

In addition, several other studies compared the recommended daily allowance (RDAs) for magnesium—420 mg for males and 320 mg for females—to the daily magnesium content from the standard diet in the United States. They concluded that half of the American population is estimated to be eating a magnesium-deficient diet which increases the risks of vitamin D deficiency and subsequent health disorders.

Since magnesium is "consumed" by the vitamin D activation process in the liver and kidneys, people with poor magnesium status and ingesting large amounts of vitamin D will develop a more dangerous magnesium deficiency.

Recommended Intakes

The Recommended Dietary Allowances (RDAs) for magnesium in the United States are: (table 6.1)

- for infants 0 to 6 months, the AI[3] is 30 mg daily
- for infants 6 to 12 months, the AI is 75 mg daily
- for 1 to 3 years old, the RDA is 80 mg daily
- for 4 to 8 years old, the RDA is 130 mg daily
- for 9 to 13 years old, the RDA is 240 mg daily
- for 14 to 18 years old male, the RDA is 410 mg daily
- for 14 to 18 years old female, the RDA is 360 mg daily
- for 14 to 18 years old pregnant female, the RDA is 400 mg daily
- for 14 to 18 years old lactating female, the RDA is 360 mg daily
- for 19 to 30 years old male, the RDA is 400 mg daily
- for 19 to 30 years old female, the RDA is 310 mg daily
- for 19 to 30 years old pregnant female, the RDA is 350 mg daily
- for 19 to 30 years old lactating female, the RDA is 310 mg daily
- for 31 to 50 years old male, the RDA is 420 mg daily
- for 31 to 50 years old female, the RDA is 320 mg daily
- for 31 to 50 years old pregnant female, the RDA is 360 mg daily
- for 31 to 50 years old lactating female, the RDA is 320 mg daily
- for 51+ years old males, the RDA is 420 mg daily
- for 51+ years old females, the RDA is 320 mg daily

table 1.6.1

How can you prevent magnesium deficiency?

Eating a balanced healthy diet containing magnesium-rich foods such as nuts, leafy green vegetables, nuts, legumes, seeds, whole grains, and foods that are high in fiber will allow you to prevent magnesium deficiency.

As all enzymes that metabolize vitamin D require magnesium, you should add to the current RDA **a magnesium supplement in the range of 150–350 mg per day when taking high doses of vitamin D.**

For example, male adults aged 31 to 50 need to get 420 mg of magnesium daily (according to the RDAs). If they are taking high doses of vitamin D, they should increase their magnesium supplementation by 250-350 mg, depending on their body weight and the amount of vitamin D they take. You can use this calculator to know the lower and upper recommended magnesium you should consume each day for optimal health outcomes.

https://www.biospherenutrition.co.nz/blogs/magnesium/how-much-magnesium-should-i-take

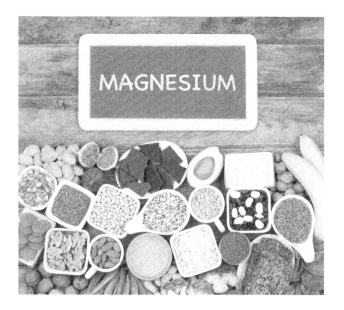

You can get this amount of magnesium from food. Some good sources of magnesium include:

- Leafy greens | serving: 1 cup | magnesium content: 157 mg
- dark chocolate (70% cocoa)| serving: 28 grams | magnesium content: 61 mg
- pumpkin seeds | serving: 28 grams | magnesium content: 150 mg
- cooked black beans | serving: 1 cup | magnesium content: 120 mg
- chia seeds | serving: 30 grams | magnesium content: 111 mg
- soymilk | serving: 1 cup | magnesium content: 63 mg
- almonds | serving: 30 grams | magnesium content: 80 mg
- spinach, boiled | serving: ½ cup | magnesium content: 78 mg
- cashews | serving: 30 grams | magnesium content: 74 mg
- dry buckwheat | serving: 28 grams | magnesium content: 65 mg
- peanuts | serving: ¼ cup | magnesium content: 63 mg
- avocado | serving: One medium avocado | magnesium content: 58 mg

- brown rice cooked | serving: ½ cup | magnesium content: 42 mg
- milk | serving: 1 cup | magnesium content: 24 mg
- salmon | serving: Half a fillet (178 grams) | magnesium content: 24 mg
- Banana | serving: one large banana | magnesium content: 40 mg

table 1.6.2

You can use this online daily supply calculator to estimate how much magnesium you are getting from the diet. https://www.biolectra.com/facts-about-magnesium/daily-supply-calculator/

Symptoms of magnesium deficiency

Magnesium deficiency can cause:

- loss of appetite
- nausea and vomiting
- numbness and tingling,
- abnormal heart rhythms and seizures
- high blood pressure
- fatigue and weakness
- muscle spasms
- hyper-excitability
- personality changes
- shaking
- pins and needles
- sleepiness

Supplements

A magnesium supplement may be required in case of low magnesium status when taking high doses of vitamin D. Magnesium supplements come in different forms, including:

- magnesium citrate (easily absorbed orally)
- magnesium chloride (easily absorbed orally)
- magnesium taurate (easily absorbed orally and suitable for high blood sugar and high blood pressure
- magnesium malate (easily absorbed orally)
- magnesium lactate (easily absorbed orally and gentler in the digestive system)
- magnesium sulfate (**poorly absorbed**)
- magnesium oxide (**poorly absorbed**)

---

1. **enzymes** are a type of protein located within a cell. Enzymes produce particular chemical reactions in the human body to help promote and sustain the body's health and integrity.
2. **hydroxylation** refers to the process that introduces a hydroxyl group [-OH] into an organic compound.
3. **adequate Intake** (AI) *is a recommended average daily intake level of a nutrient,* expected to satisfy or exceed the amount required to maintain a specified nutritional state or criterion of adequacy in practically all members of a specific healthy group.

6

WHY VITAMIN K2 IS IMPORTANT?

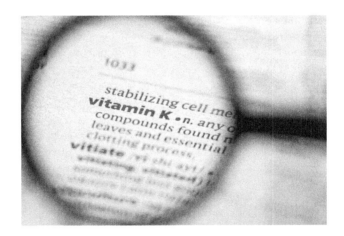

Increased levels of vitamin D3 require increased levels of vitamin K, specifically vitamin K2 (menaquinone). Without the right amount of vitamin K2, high doses of vitamin D supplementation may not be as effective as they would be. Vitamin D and K2 work together synergetically to optimize calcium metabolism, promote bone health and prevent coronary artery disease. Vitamin K2 guides calcium — ingested from diet or supplementation— to bones and prevents its absorption into organs, arteries, and joint spaces.

Vitamin K is known for its beneficial effects on blood coagulation. Vitamin K is required by the liver to make several factors necessary for blood to clot correctly. The role of vitamin K in regulating the healthy function of calcium has only recently been identified. Vitamin K2 has now been found to exert its effect as an essential cofactor in calcium metabolism, guiding calcium —ingested from diet or supplementation— to bones and preventing its absorption into organs, arteries, and joint spaces. Without the action of vitamin K2, the regulation of calcium concentration will be severely affected in various tissues.

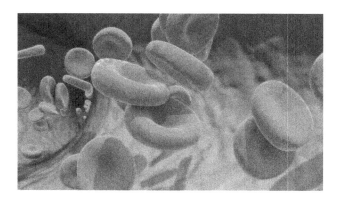

Vitamin K2 (MK-4 and MK-7)

Vitamin K, the generic name given to a group of fat-soluble vitamins with a similar chemical structure, is naturally present in some foods and available as a dietary supplement. The lactic acid bacteria also produce some vitamin K2 in our intestines.

Vitamin K exists naturally as phylloquinone (vitamin K1) and a group of menaquinone (vitamin K2)—each of these forms has very different contributions to human health. However, many studies have reported better health benefits with vitamin K2 than vitamin K1.

Vitamin K1 (phylloquinone) is the primary dietary source of vitamin

K, accounting for roughly 90% of total vitamin K intakes. It is found in green leafy vegetables like kale, broccoli, green salads, spinach, olive oil, and soybean oil. However, the absorption of vitamin K1 from food sources is poor, about 20%.

Vitamin K2 comprises a group of molecules that differ in side chains' length. The most important forms of vitamin K2 are MK-4 and MK-7. Both are found in animal products such as meat, dairy, eggs, cheese, yogurt, liver, natto, butter, egg yolks, and fermented soybeans.

The market adopted vitamin K2 in its menaquinone-4 (MK-4) and menaquinone-7 (MK-7) forms as dietary supplements. However, with a better understanding of the value of MK-7 over MK-4, MK-7 becomes the ingredient of choice as a nutritional supplement. Several studies demonstrated that a nutritional intake of MK-7 is well absorbed in humans and substantially raises serum MK-7 levels, whereas MK-4 does not affect serum MK-4 levels.

Health benefits of Vitamin K2

A growing body of evidence supports that besides its role in blood clotting and bone metabolism, Vitamin K exerts beneficial anti-calcification, anti-cancer, bone-forming, and insulin-sensitizing actions.

A good vitamin K status is associated with a myriad of health benefits, including prevention and treatment of arterial calcifications, improvements in bone health, especially osteoporosis, enhancement in insulin sensitivity, and prevention of certain cancers. Vitamin K1 is mainly involved in blood coagulation, whereas vitamin K2 has a more diverse range of functions in the body.

Vitamin K2 is known to function as a coagulant, and its deficit can have severe consequences. Vitamin K2 also effectively reduces the calcium levels available in the blood, thus decreasing the calcium deposit in vascular structures and improving bone strength. In addition, It exerts beneficial effects on insulin sensitivity, blood vessel elasticity, cardiovascular diseases, and cancer prevention.

Vitamin K2 and Vitamin D

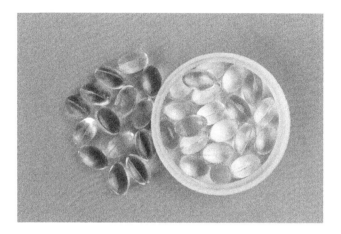

Emerging scientific and clinical literature currently exists for vitamin D and vitamin K2 due to the increasing awareness concerning the role of cofactors in vitamin D adequacy. PUBMED (The National Library of Medicine, and the first source for biomedical literature) lists ≥ 1,067 publications using the keywords **"vitamin D"** and **"vitamin K"** in either the title or abstract from 1938 to the present, with most of the research published in the last two decades. This total includes publications that combine the use of one of the following terms with vitamin D:

- vitamin k supplementation (≥ 211 publications),
- vitamin k2 (≥ 198 publications),
- vitamin k deficiency (≥ publications).

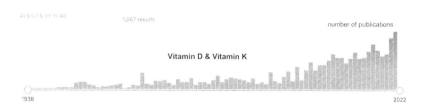

figure 1.6.1: increase in the number of articles published with the term magnesium and vitamin D in the title or abstract (in PUBMED.)

Vitamin K2 (menaquinone) is an essential cofactor for vitamin D. Without the right amount of vitamin K2, a high-dose vitamin D supplementation may not be as effective as it would be. Vitamin D and vitamin K2 have a synergetic action and should be taken together.

Many clinical and epidemiological studies have established that vitamin D and K2 work together synergetically to optimize calcium metabolism, promote bone health and prevent coronary artery disease. Vitamin K2, through its carboxylation of osteocalcin, guides calcium —ingested from diet or supplementation— to bones and prevents its absorption into organs, arteries, and joint spaces.

Recommended Intakes

The Recommended Dietary Allowances (RDAs) for vitamin k in the United States are:

- for infants 0 to 6 months, the AI is 2.0 mcg daily
- for infants 6 to 12 months, the AI is 2.5 mcg daily
- for 1 to 3 years old male, the RDA is 30 mcg daily
- for 1 to 3 years old female, the RDA is 30 mcg daily
- for 4 to 8 years old, male the RDA is 55 mcg daily
- for 4 to 8 years old, female the RDA is 55 mcg daily
- for 9 to 13 years old, male the RDA is 60 mcg daily
- for 9 to 13 years old, female the RDA is 60 mcg daily
- for 14 to 18 years old male, the RDA is 75 mcg daily
- for 14 to 18 years old female, the RDA is 75 mcg daily
- for 14 to 18 years old pregnant female, the RDA is 75 mcg daily
- for 14 to 18 years old lactating female, the RDA is 75 mcg daily
- for 19+ years old male, the RDA is 120 mcg daily

- for 19+ years old female, the RDA is 90 mcg daily
- for 19+ years old pregnant female, the RDA is 90 mcg daily
- for 19+ years old lactating female, the RDA is 90 mcg daily

table 1.6.1

Vitamin K2 and Vitamin D supplementation

Increased levels of vitamin D3 require increased levels of vitamin K, specifically vitamin K2 (menaquinone). Without the right amount of vitamin K2, a high-dose vitamin D supplementation may not be as effective as it would be. Vitamin D and K2 work together synergetically to optimize calcium metabolism, promote bone health and prevent coronary artery disease. Vitamin K2 guides calcium — ingested from diet or supplementation— to bones and prevents absorption into organs, arteries, and joint spaces.

Thus, like for magnesium, most people need to increase the amount of vitamin k2 they typically consume. Table I.7.2 below is given as a reference to see the relationship between vitamin D and associated vitamin K2 daily intakes and estimate your daily needs of vitamin K2.

It indicates the daily maintenance doses to take to keep the vitamin D [25(OH)D] blood levels at 40 nanograms/mL (after the fill-up period). Supplementation to achieve optimum Vitamin D levels is considered adequate for overall health.

- for 50 kg body weight and **4,500 IU** daily vitamin D3 supplementation; the vitamin K2 supplementation is **200 mcg** daily
- for 55 kg body weight and **4,950** IU daily vitamin D3 supplementation; the vitamin K2 supplementation is **220 mcg** daily

- for 60 kg body weight and **5,400 IU** daily vitamin D3 supplementation; the vitamin K2 supplementation is **240** mcg daily
- for 65 kg body weight and **5,850 IU** daily vitamin D3 supplementation; the vitamin K2 supplementation is **260** mcg daily
- for 70 kg body weight and **6,300 IU** daily vitamin D3 supplementation; the vitamin K2 supplementation is **280** mcg daily
- for 75 kg body weight and **6,750 IU** daily vitamin D3 supplementation; the vitamin K2 supplementation is **300** mcg daily
- for 80 kg body weight and **7,200 IU** daily vitamin D3 supplementation; the vitamin K2 supplementation is **320** mcg daily
- for 85 kg body weight and **7,650 IU** daily vitamin D3 supplementation; the vitamin K2 supplementation is **340** mcg daily
- for 90 kg body weight and **8,100 IU** daily vitamin D3 supplementation; the vitamin K2 supplementation is **360** mcg daily
- for 95 kg body weight and **8,550 IU** daily vitamin D3 supplementation; the vitamin K2 supplementation is **380** mcg daily
- for 100 kg body weight and **9,000 IU** daily vitamin D3 supplementation; the vitamin K2 supplementation is **400** mcg daily
- for 105 kg body weight and **9,450 IU** daily vitamin D3 supplementation; the vitamin K2 supplementation is **420** mcg daily
- for 110 kg body weight and **9,900 IU** daily vitamin D3 supplementation; the vitamin K2 supplementation is **440** mcg daily

table 1.6.2

Adequate doses of both vitamin D and vitamin K2 (MK-7) are needed to raise and maintain the vitamin D [25(OH)D] levels in the optimal range of 40 to 60 nanograms/mL (100 to 150 nmol/L).

So you have to increase your intake of vitamin k2-rich foods or dietary supplements.

How can you get enough vitamin K2?

Eating a balanced diet containing vitamin K2-rich foods will allow you to get sufficient amounts. Some good sources of vitamin K2 include: (table 7.3)

- Natto | serving: 100 grams | Vitamin K2 content: 1104 mcg
- Kale, cooked | serving: 100 grams | Vitamin K2 content: 817 mcg
- Mustard Greens, cooked | serving: 100 grams | Vitamin K2 content: 593 mcg
- Collard Greens, cooked | serving: 100 grams | Vitamin K2 content: 407 mcg
- Swiss Chard | serving: 100 grams | Vitamin K2 content: 830 mcg
- Broccoli, cooked | serving: 100 grams | Vitamin K2 content: 141 mcg

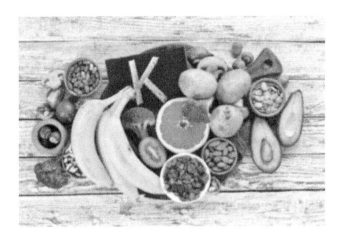

- Egg Yolk | serving: 100 grams | magnesium content: 16 mg
- Hard cheeses | serving: 100 grams | Vitamin K2 content: 77 mg
- Beef Liver | serving: 100 grams | Vitamin K2 content: 106 mcg
- Pork Chops | serving: 100 grams | Vitamin K2 content: 70 mg
- Chicken | serving: 100 grams | Vitamin K2 content: 60 mcg
- Goose liver | serving: 100 grams | Vitamin K2 content: 369 mg
- Black Bean Natto | serving: 100 grams | Vitamin K2 content: 798 mcg
- Pepperoni | serving: 100 grams | Vitamin K2 content: 42 mcg
- Salami | serving: 1 cup | Vitamin K2 content: 24 mg
- Butter | serving: 100 grams | Vitamin K2 content: 21 mcg
- Chicken wings | serving: 100 grams | Vitamin K2 content: 25.3 mg

table 1.6.3

7

WHY CALCIUM IS IMPORTANT?

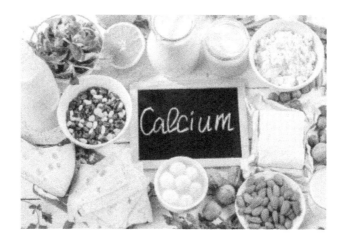

Calcium is strongly associated with many beneficial roles that vitamin D plays in the human body. Calcium is essential for building strong and healthy bones. Calcium is also necessary for many physiological functions, including muscle contractions, hormone secretion, and the normal functioning of many enzymes. Calcium deficiency can cause rickets in children and many bone disorders in adults, although these conditions are more generally caused by low vitamin D status.

Calcium is the most abundant mineral and the fifth most abundant element in the body. Almost all (99%) calcium in the body is stored in the bone as hydroxyapatite, which provides skeletal strength. The remaining 1% is contained in the blood, muscle, and other tissues. Approximately half of that (the ionic fraction that is physiologically active) is free in the blood.

This fraction of calcium plays a crucial role in many body's physiological processes, including skeletal mineralization, muscle contractions, neural impulses transmission, blood clotting/coagulation, hormone secretion, and the normal functioning of many enzymes.

In order to perform these critical daily functions, the body works to keep a stable amount of calcium in the blood and tissues. Blood calcium concentrations are maintained within a range of 8.5–10.5 mg/dL (2.2–2.7 mmol/L).

The human body doesn't produce calcium, so diet is the only way to get calcium. The body adjusts the amount of calcium in cells and blood tightly and takes calcium from the bones and teeth when needed to maintain a normal calcium level in the blood.

Three molecules regulate the amount of calcium in the blood: calcitriol (the active form of vitamin D), parathyroid hormone (PTH), and calcitonin hormone. Calcitriol is produced in the kidneys, parathyroid hormone (PTH) is released by the parathyroid glands, and the thyroid glands secrete calcitonin.

If calcium concentrations drop too low in the blood, parathyroid hormone (PTH) will signal the bones to secrete calcium into the blood. The PTH also stimulates vitamin D production in the kidneys and thus indirectly improves the absorption of calcium in the intestines. At the same time, PTH signals the kidneys to secrete less calcium in the urine.

As serum calcium concentrations rise, the release of parathyroid hormone (PTH) decreases to keep a healthy calcium status.

When blood calcium levels become too high, PTH secretes calcitonin, which functions to maintain calcium levels in the normal range. Calcitonin reduces calcium concentrations in the blood by inhibiting the release of calcium from bones, reducing calcium absorption in the intestine, and signaling the kidneys to reabsorb less calcium, resulting in more significant amounts of calcium eliminated in the urine.

Vitamin D

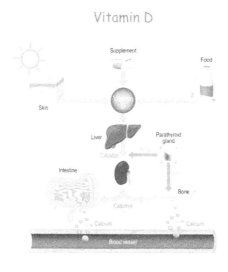

An enormous and growing scientific and clinical literature currently exists for vitamin D and calcium. PUBMED (The National Library of Medicine, and the first source for biomedical literature) lists ≥ 33,521

publications using the keywords **"vitamin D"** and **"calcium"** in either the title or abstract from 1928 to the present, with most of the research published in the last four decades. This total includes publications that combine the use of one of the following terms with vitamin D:

- calcium bone (≥ 16,512 publications),
- calcium deficiency (≥9,288 publications),
- calcium osteoporosis (≥ 7,023 publications),
- calcium absorption (≥ 3,456 publications),
- calcium magnesium (≥ 1,963 publications).

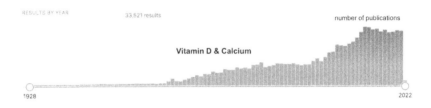

figure 3.1.1: increase in the number of articles published with the term "calcium" and "vitamin D" in the title or abstract (in PUBMED.)

Calcium Deficiency

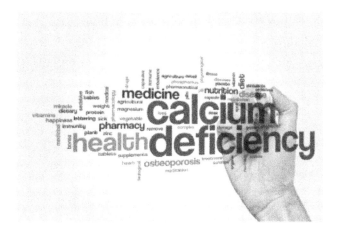

Calcium deficiency, also known as hypocalcemia, is characterized by a serum calcium level below 8.5 mg/dL (2.12 mmol/L) or an ionized calcium level less than 4.61 mg/dL (1.15 mmol/L). Calcium deficiency may cause no short-term symptoms because the body keeps and regulates calcium levels by taking it directly from the bones and teeth. However, symptoms will develop as the disorder progresses, and long-term impacts can be severe, including dental changes, osteomalacia, rickets, cataracts, alterations in the brain, and osteoporosis.

What causes calcium inadequacy?

- Calcium inadequacy may be due to several factors, including:
- insufficient calcium intake over a prolonged period
- drugs that may reduce calcium absorption (e.g. Bisphosphonates, Sensipar, Phenytoin)
- food intolerance to meals rich in calcium
- hormonal modifications (e.g. menopause, pregnancy)

The consequence of vitamin D deficiency

Calcitriol sustains calcium balance through its actions in the intestines, kidneys, bones, and parathyroid glands. A vitamin D deficiency means the body can't produce enough calcitriol, which leads to poor calcium absorption from the diet. And consequently, the body takes calcium from the skeleton, weakening the bone and preventing strong, new bone formation.

Recommended Intakes

The Recommended Dietary Allowances (RDAs) for calcium set by the National Academy of Medicine in 2010:

- for infants 0 to 6 months, the RDA is 200 mg daily
- for infants 6 to 12 months, the RDA is 260 mg daily
- for 1 to 3 years old, the RDA is 700 mg daily
- for 4 to 8 years old, the RDA is 1,000 mg daily
- for 9 to 13 years old, the RDA is 1,300 mg daily
- for 14 to 18 years old, the RDA is 1,300 mg daily
- for 19 to 30 years old, the RDA is 1,000 mg daily
- for 31 to 50 years old, the RDA is 1,000 mg daily
- for 51 to 70 years old males, the RDA is 1,000 mg daily
- for 51 to 70 years old females, the RDA is 1,200 mg daily
- for 70+ years old, the RDA is 1,200 mg daily
- for 14 to 18 years old, pregnant or lactating, the RDA is 1,300 mg.
- for 19 to 50 years old, pregnant or lactating, the RDA is 1,000 mg.

How can you get enough calcium?

Calcium is essential for many physiological functions, including skeletal mineralization, muscle contractions, hormone secretion, and the normal functioning of many enzymes. Calcium must be taken from natural sources or nutritional supplements. Calcium is available in dairy products and several nondairy products, including grains, green leafy vegetables, sardines, salmon, and fortified foods.

While taking calcium supplements may induce adverse effects, meeting your calcium requirements through your diet is feasible if you make the necessary efforts. If you don't have sufficient calcium in your diet, you should consider taking low-dose calcium supplements to fill the gap.

Some good sources of calcium include:

- Yogurt, plain, nonfat | Serving: 8 ounces | Calories: 137 | Calcium(mg): 488
- Yogurt, plain, low fat | Serving: 8 ounces | Calories: 154 | Calcium(mg): 448
- Milk, low fat (1 %) | Serving: 1 cup | Calories: 102 | Calcium(mg): 305
- Soy milk, unsweetened | Serving: 8 ounces | Calories: 80 | Calcium(mg): 301
- Yogurt, soy, plain | Serving: 1 cup | Calories: 150 | Calcium(mg): 300
- Milk, fat free (skim) | Serving: 1 cup | Calories: 83 | Calcium(mg): 298
- Buttermilk, low fat | Serving: 1 cup | Calories: 98 | Calcium(mg): 284
- Yogurt, Greek, plain, low fat | Serving: 8 ounces | Calories: 166 | Calcium(mg): 261
- Yogurt, Greek, plain, nonfat | Serving: 8 ounces | Calories: 134 | Calcium(mg): 250
- Parmesan cheese | Serving: 28 grams | Calories: 120 | Calcium(mg): 242
- Lambsquarters, raw | Serving: 100 grams | Calories: 43 | Calcium(mg): 309

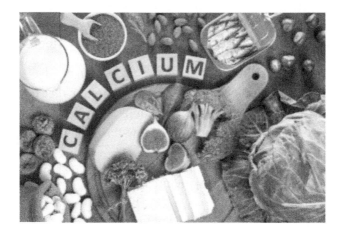

- Nettles, cooked | Serving: 1 cup | Calories: 37 | Calcium(mg): 428
- Mustard spinach, cooked | Serving: 1 cup | Calories: 29 | Calcium(mg): 284
- Amaranth leaves, cooked | Serving: 1 cup | Calories: 28 | Calcium(mg): 276
- Collard greens, cooked | Serving: 1 cup | Calories: 63 | Calcium(mg): 268
- Spinach, cooked | Serving: 1 cup | Calories: 41 | Calcium(mg): 245
- Turnip greens, cooked | Serving: 1 cup | Calories: 29 | Calcium(mg): 197
- Kale, cooked | Serving: 1 cup | Calories: 43 | Calcium(mg): 177
- Sardines, canned | Serving: 3 ounces | Calories: 177 | Calcium(mg): 325
- Salmon, canned, solids with bone | Serving: 3 ounces | Calories: 118 | Calcium(mg): 181
- Tahini (sesame butter or paste) | Serving: 1 tablespoon | Calories: 94 | Calcium(mg): 154
- Grapefruit juice, 100%, fortified | Serving: 1 cup | Calories: 94 | Calcium(mg): 350
- Orange juice, 100%, fortified | Serving: 1 cup | Calories: 117 | Calcium(mg): 349

- Almond milk, unsweetened | Serving: 1 cup | Calories: 36 | Calcium(mg): 442

Types of Calcium Supplements

The two primary forms of calcium are calcium carbonate and calcium citrate. Each has benefits and inconveniences. Calcium carbonate supplements are the cheapest and usually an excellent practical option because they contain the highest elemental calcium (nearly 40% by weight), whereas calcium citrate has only 21% of elemental calcium.

However, calcium carbonate requires stomach acid in the intestine, generated with food in the stomach. Therefore, people taking carbonate calcium should take it with meals to increase calcium absorption. In contrast, calcium citrate is absorbed more efficiently than calcium carbonate and taken on an empty stomach.

8

VITAMIN D TOXICITY

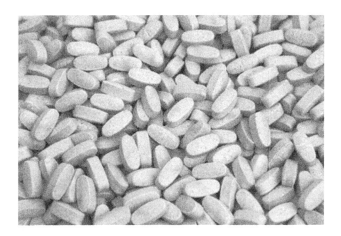

Strong evidence shows that vitamin D toxicity is one of the extremely rarest medical conditions and is typically due to deliberate or accidental intake of extremely high doses. Doses of more than 50,000 international units (IU) per day increase levels of circulating vitamin D [25(OH)D] to more than 150 nanograms/mL (375 nmol/L) and may be associated with hypercalcemia.

The maximum amount of vitamin D healthy adults can take safely every day has not been established. Several government agencies consider the Upper Intake Level (UL) of 4,000 IU (100 mcg) per day as safe for regular use, despite evidence of the safety of 10,000 IU (250 mcg) per day.

Vitamin D overdosing, also called hypervitaminosis D, is extremely rare and only occurs with prolonged consumption of 40,000 to 50,000 international units of vitamin D3 per day. This health condition is called hypercalcemia and traduces a very high calcium concentration (higher than 11 mg/dl or 2.75 mmol/l).

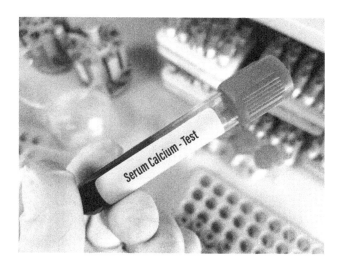

Calcium levels in the blood are kept within a limited range due to the central role of calcium in normal body function. Calcium is essential in normal cell function, including muscle function, nerve transmission, bone structure, hormone action, and blood clotting. When calcium levels become high, people experience symptoms affecting the stomach and intestines, such as nausea, vomiting, and loss of appetite. Severe hypercalcemia may cause serious conditions such as kidney stones and calcifications in the organs.

Untreated hypercalcemia can cause kidney failure and, in extreme cases, death. The most common causes of hypercalcemia are malignancy, sarcoidosis, and primary hyperparathyroidism.

Much scientific and clinical literature on "**vitamin D and toxicity**" currently exists. PUBMED (The National Library of Medicine, and the first source for biomedical literature) lists

- ≥ 2,611 publications that use the term *vitamin D* and toxicity,
- ≥ 2,251 publications that use the term *vitamin D* and toxicity in either the title or abstract from 1932 to the present, with most of the studies published in the last four decades.

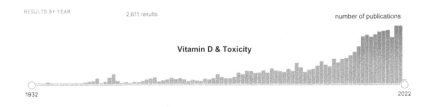

Recent clinical studies concluded that most patients with very high vitamin D levels—25(OH)D levels > 150 nanograms/mL—have normal serum calcium. However, at such levels, the risk of severe hypercalcemia may increase. Treatment involves stopping vitamin D, reducing dietary calcium, restoring blood volume, and administering corticosteroids or bisphosphonates if necessary.

Several studies have been conducted to assess the safety of vitamin D supplementation at various dose levels.

- in healthy individuals, no adverse outcomes were reported giving 836 IU per day, 5,500 IU per day, or 11,000 IU per day during five months.
- a daily intake of 10,000 IU of vitamin D over prolonged

periods did not cause toxicity, even when individuals received significant solar-UVB exposure to bare skin.
- the vitamin D administration at 1000 mcg (40,000 IU) per day induces toxic effects in the infant within 1 to 4 months. In adults, administration of 1250 mcg (50,000 IU) per day for several months can lead to intoxication.

However, suppose you suffer from a severe vitamin D deficiency. In that case, your doctor may prescribe therapy with a daily intake of 60,000 IU to fill your body's store for 2-4 weeks without any adverse effects.

Vitamin D intoxication is one of the rarest medical conditions. Intoxicated people show a variety of symptoms, including:

- nausea and vomiting
- fatigue and weakness
- loss of appetite
- aches
- cardiac arrhythmia
- headache

Does sunlight combined with supplementation lead to vitamin D overdose?

To understand the safety of regular vitamin D supplementation at high doses of up to 10,000 IU, you must know that vitamin D3 production in the skin with total body exposure to the sun is comparable to taking an oral dose between 250—625 mcg (10,000—25,000 IU) per day.

During prolonged sunlight exposure, when the concentration of vitamin D precursors formed in the skin reaches a specific level, relevant regulatory mechanisms in your body function to degrade the excessive production of vitamin D3 and prevent toxic levels. **We can consider this natural, safe level of 25,000 IU (625 mcg) as a threshold.**

During the summer months, for example, people who consume 10,000 International Units of the vitamin D3 per day, and get long daily sunbaths with total body exposure, can reach a level of 500—750 mcg (20,000—30,000 IU).

Therefore, excessive daily exposure to sun rays combined with supplementation of 10,000 IU per day can lead to exceeding the natural threshold of 25,000 IU (625 mcg). In this case, they may reduce their dietary intake or sun exposure.

If you're regularly taking a very high dose of vitamin D as a supplement. If you worry about toxicity, get your blood calcium level tested. As long as the serum calcium level stays normal, you are safe.

PART II

PART II

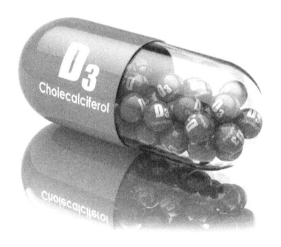

9

THE VITAMIN D DEFICIENCY PANDEMIC

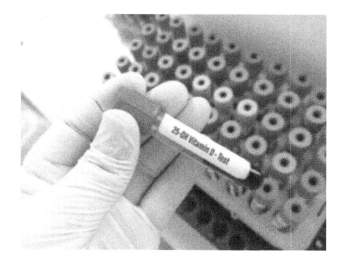

"" Although there are several areas of debate concerning vitamin D requirements and the effect of vitamin D intake and status on human health, there is a consensus that preventing vitamin D deficiency is a public health priority. Vitamin D deficiency is strongly correlated with an excess of mortality of roughly 28%, all causes combined and influences myriad health outcomes.

With more than a billion people vitamin D deficient worldwide, Vitamin D deficiency continues to evolve into a global public health problem. Vitamin D deficiency happens when one or both of the following factors exists: the total daily intakes are lower than the amount adequate for maintaining health, exposure to sunlight is poor, kidneys cannot activate vitamin D to calcitriol, or absorption of vitamin D from the digestive system is deficient. Vitamin D deficiency and insufficiency appear to be pandemic problems and are more frequent in high-latitude inhabitants than in low-latitude areas.

In the last decades, vitamin D deficiency has again become a major public health interest due to its association with poor health outcomes such as bone disorders (osteoporosis, osteomalacia, fractures), and more recently with the association of adequate levels of vitamin D in preventing cancers, diabetes type 2, heart disease, kidney and liver diseases, nervous system disorders and other chronic illnesses.

There is a huge and growing body of scientific literature and clinical studies for vitamin D deficiency. PUBMED (National Library of Medicine) lists ≥ 35,973 publications using the keyword "**vitamin D deficiency**" in either the title or abstract from 1945 to the present. This total includes articles that combine the use of vitamin D deficiency with one of the following terms:

- adults (≥ 15,050 articles)
- bone (≥ 13,586 articles),
- older adults (≥ 11,634 articles),
- health (≥ 9,696 articles),
- children (≥ 7,805 articles),
- chronic diseases (≥ 6,359 articles),

- cancer (≥ 3,541 articles),
- women (≥ 4,724 articles),
- cancer (≥ 3,541 articles)
- diabetes (≥ 3,433 articles),
- pregnancy (≥ 2,335 articles),
- obesity (≥1,893 articles),
- immune (≥1,824),
- inflammatory (≥ 1,551 articles),
- depression (≥630 articles).

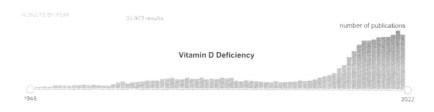

figure 1.1: increase in the number of articles published with the term "vitamin D deficiency" in the title or abstract (in PUBMED.)

In children, vitamin D deficiency causes rickets, a severe skeletal disorder characterized by the failure of bone tissue to become correctly mineralized. Rickets was a common severe skeletal disease that affected children from the seventieth century to the early 20th century. Still, it mostly disappeared during the early 20th century after discovering vitamin D and its production in the skin through sunlight exposure. Foods including milk were irradiated by ultraviolet light or fortified with vitamin D.

Children and people who were vitamin D deficient absorbed only about 10—15 percent of their daily recommended allowance (RDAs) of calcium and 60 percent of their RDAs of phosphorus. When vitamin D deficiency gets corrected, active vitamin D helps optimize intestinal calcium absorption (30—40 percent increase) and phos-phorus absorption (about 80 percent increase). Vitamin D, thus treated and prevented rickets and osteomalacia.

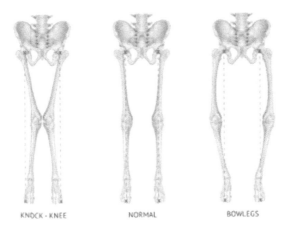

KNOCK - KNEE   NORMAL   BOWLEGS

Rickets initiated studies that led to the discovery of vitamin D itself in the twentieth century. Without the vitamin D produced from the sun or ingested via diet or nutritional supplementation, childs' bones could not obtain the calcium they require to be strong.

In adults, vitamin D deficiency/insufficiency is associated with an increased risk of developing chronic inflammatory diseases, cardio-vascular diseases, bone disorders, kidney and liver conditions, autoimmune diseases, neurological diseases, cancers, and diabetes. Low vitamin D status is also linked to morbidity and mortality, disease severity and symptoms worsening.

Groups at Risk of Vitamin D Deficiency

For many people, eating a balanced and vitamin D-rich diet and exposing themselves to sunlight may maintain an adequate vitamin D status in the spring and summer months. People who live above the 37-degree latitude line get little to no UVB exposure between the autumn and winter months to make vitamin D and need dietary supplements to meet their minimal vitamin D requirements (associated with bone health).

However, individuals with:

- residence latitude above the line of the 35th parallel in the northern hemisphere,
- poor physical activity,
- limited sunlight exposure,
- obesity (current studies suggested that vitamin D deficiency is 35 percent higher in obese people irrespective of residence latitude and age),
- dark skin (current studies showed that individuals with higher-skin-melanin content or using extensive skin coverages are more likely to develop vitamin D deficiency)
- nursing home residents (50—60 percent of nursing home residents had vitamin D deficiency In the United States, according to a number of studies),
- advanced age (In the United States, studies found that 61 percent of the elderly population are vitamin D deficient, according to recent studies)
- unbalanced diet,
- kidney diseases,
- conditions that limit fat absorption,
- malabsorption syndrome,
- liver disease,
- and other comorbid illnesses

must take a daily vitamin D supplement all year round to correct their vitamin D status.

Health effects of vitamin D deficiency

Vitamin D is a hormone that targets distant tissues where it produces multiple beneficial effects and contributes to numerous metabolic functions. Vitamin D receptor (VDR) proteins that allow the body to respond to vitamin D are present in the heart, brain, lung, skin, pancreas, parathyroid gland, thyroid gland, and more than 400 tissues and cell types and almost everywhere in the body. Consequently, active Vitamin D targets thousands of genes and is associated with overall health outcomes. Higher circulating vitamin D [25(OH)D] levels have been associated with a decrease in risk for a growing list of chronic diseases that include cardiovascular diseases, autoimmune diseases, bone disorders, inflammatory conditions, cognitive decline, osteoporosis, multiple sclerosis, psoriasis, and various cancers

VITAMIN D deficiency

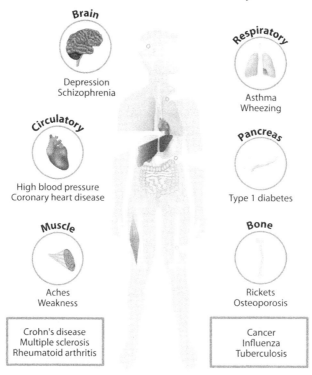

Brain

Depression
Schizophrenia

Respiratory

Asthma
Wheezing

Circulatory

High blood pressure
Coronary heart disease

Pancreas

Type 1 diabetes

Muscle

Aches
Weakness

Bone

Rickets
Osteoporosis

Crohn's disease
Multiple sclerosis
Rheumatoid arthritis

Cancer
Influenza
Tuberculosis

Conversely, low vitamin D status is associated with a growing list of several risk factors for poor health outcomes, decreased energy and activity, altered health, and more susceptibility to illnesses.

Achieving adequate vitamin D status will improve your overall health by protecting you from conditions associated with vitamin D deficiency and possibly helping to treat them. This include:

Certain types of cancers such as colon, breast, ovarian, and prostate cancers. Recent clinical studies have pointed out the role of Vitamin D in cell growth and proliferation, suggesting it can affect the instigation of cancer by interrupting the formation of cancer cells. Vitamin D may have beneficial effects in preventing the development of certain cancers and lowering their incidence, particularly when the total vitamin D [25(OH)D] level is more than **50 nanograms/mL (125 nmol/L).**

Cardiovascular diseases. Published studies have suggested vitamin D deficiency is associated with heart failure, heart attacks, strokes, peripheral arterial disease, and high blood pressure. Vitamin D may have beneficial effects in preventing and reducing the incidence of cardiovascular diseases, particularly when the total vitamin D [25(OH)D] level is more than 40 nanograms/mL.

Type 1 diabetes, type 2 diabetes. Clinical studies have pointed to the positive preventive relationship between vitamin D and type 2 diabetes and the association between vitamin D supplementation and type 1 diabetes. Vitamin D has beneficial effects in preventing and lowering the severity of type 1 and type 2 diabetes, particularly when the total vitamin D [25(OH)D] level is more than 40 nanograms/mL.

Infections and disorders of the immune system. Recent studies and epidemiological data have indicated that vitamin D deficiency is positively correlated with the exacerbation of inflammatory autoimmune diseases and infectious diseases, such as rheumatoid arthritis, flu, and multiple sclerosis. Calcitriol, the active form of vitamin D directly affects immune cells, playing a key role in autoimmune diseases. Vitamin D has beneficial effects in preventing and lowering the incidence and risks associated with infections and disorders of the immune system, particularly when the total vitamin D [25(OH)D] level is more than 40 nanograms/mL.

Bone diseases, falls, and fractures in the elderly. Vitamin D inadequacy is prevalent in the elderly due to various risk factors, including reduced sunlight exposure, deficient intestinal absorption, and impaired vitamin D activation in the liver and kidneys. Vitamin D inadequacy is prevalent in the elderly due to various risk factors, including reduced sunlight exposure, deficient intestinal absorption, and impaired vitamin D activation in the liver and kidneys. Vitamin D supplementation results in positive outcomes concerning fall prevention, particularly when patients reach and maintain a total vitamin D [25(OH)D] level of more than 40 nanograms/mL.

Weight gain and obesity. It is suggested that the concentration of 25(OH)D is negatively correlated with the body mass index (BMI) and the percentage of fat mass. Vitamin D supplementation results in positive outcomes regarding weight gain and obesity, particularly when patients reach and maintain the total vitamin D [25(OH)D] level of more than 40 nanograms/mL.

Dementia, schizophrenia, and depression. Evidence from clinical studies has supported the association of vitamin D deficiency with many mental disorders, including schizophrenia and depression. Ongoing studies are conducted to bring more proof and support the potentially positive role of vitamin D in schizophrenia and depression treatments.

Pulmonary diseases (including COPD, and cystic fibrosis). Adequate vitamin D status has been recently associated with a decrease in severe respiratory diseases.

Autoimmune diseases. Vitamin D deficiency is linked to the development of some autoimmune diseases such as type 1 diabetes, rheumatoid arthritis, thyrotoxicosis, Crohn's disease, psoriasis, ulcerative colitis, and polymyalgia. Vitamin D has beneficial effects in preventing and lowering the incidence and risks associated with infections and disorders of the immune system, particularly when the total vitamin D [25(OH)D] level is more than 40 nanograms/mL.

Parathyroid disorders. The association between vitamin D and the parathyroid hormone (PTH) was established by several studies due to its importance in bone remodeling in the elderly. Vitamin D-deficient patients were those who had higher values of PTH, while individuals with an adequate vitamin D status had low PTH values.

Thyroid disorders. Several clinical studies have found a low vitamin D status in autoimmune thyroid diseases (AITD), showing an association between low vitamin D [25(OH)D] and the development of thyroid autoimmunity in adults.

Allergies. Observational studies have established that vitamin D deficiency may contribute to the development and/or severity of asthma and allergic diseases. It is believed that a vitamin D [25(OH)D] level in the range of 40-60 nanograms/mL may be beneficial in the prevention of asthma and allergic diseases and the reduction of their incidence.

Rheumatoid arthritis. Vitamin D deficiency has been associated with the pathogenesis of some autoimmune diseases, such as type 1 diabetes and rheumatoid arthritis.

Psoriasis. Vitamin D deficiency is linked to the development of autoimmune diseases such as psoriasis. Vitamin D has beneficial effects in preventing and lowering the incidence and risks associated with infections and disorders of the immune system, particularly when the total vitamin D [25(OH)D] level is more than 40 nanograms/mL.

Thyroid disorders. Current observational studies have suggested that deficiency of vitamin D and calcium levels were associated with the degree and severity of hypothyroidism. A vitamin D supplementation may alleviate symptoms and severity of thyroid disorders.

Cognitive decline. Recent studies have established that low serum vitamin D levels are associated with a higher risk of cognitive decline.

Fibromyalgia. Vitamin D deficiency and insufficiency have been associated with fibromyalgia. The vitamin D [25(OH)D] levels in the range of 40-60 ng/ml seem to improve disease symptoms in patients with fibromyalgia.

Multiple sclerosis. Vitamin D deficiency has been associated with the pathogenesis of autoimmune diseases, such as multiple sclerosis. Smaller vitamin D intake has been correlated with higher suscepti-bility to the development of multiple sclerosis.

Vision disorders. A growing body of evidence points to the associa-tion between vision disorders and vitamin D deficiency.

Autism spectrum disorders. Vitamin D may have beneficial outcomes in autism spectrum disorders subjects, particularly when the total vitamin D [25(OH)D] level is more than 40 nanograms/mL.

Acne. Some studies have shown that patients with acne vulgaris have lower serum vitamin D levels than vitamin D levels in healthy controls.

Chronic fatigue

Polycystic ovary syndrome (PCOS)

Chronic muscle pain

Joint and back pain

Migraines

Inflammatory bowel disease

10

KEY ROLES OF VITAMIN D

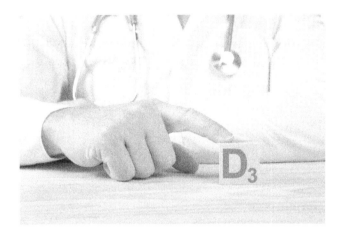

" Higher circulating vitamin D [25(OH)D] levels have been linked with a substantial reduction in risk for a long list of long-latency conditions that include bone disorders, cardiovascular diseases, autoimmune diseases, pulmonary diseases, kidneys diseases, obesity, parathyroid and thyroid disorders, type 1 and 2 diabetes, breast, prostate, colorectal cancers, cognitive decline.

For many years, vitamin D has long been known for its beneficial effects on promoting calcium and phosphorus metabolism. However, with the discovery of vitamin D receptors in various tissues and cells, many biological roles of vitamin D have been identified. In fact, researchers have identified more than 36 target organs (table 2.2.1) in which the vitamin D receptor (VDR) is present, allowing them to be susceptible to hormonally active vitamin D actions and effects. It is then believed with a high degree of confidence that vitamin D is critical for the optimal functioning of most of the body's organs where vitamin D receptors are located. Those organs are:

1. Adipose
2. Adrenal
3. Bone
4. Bone marrow
5. Brain
6. Breast
7. Cancer cells
8. Cartilage
9. Colon
10. Dendritic cells
11. Eggshell gland
12. Endothelial cells
13. Epididymis
14. Hair follicle
15. Intestine
16. Kidney
17. Liver (fetal)
18. Lung
19. Lymphocytes (B & T)
20. Mammary, breast
21. Muscle, cardiac
22. Muscle, embryonic

23. Muscle, smooth
24. Osteoblast
25. Ovary
26. Pancreas β cell
27. Pancreatic islets
28. Parathyroid
29. Parathyroid glands
30. Parotid
31. Pituitary
32. Placenta
33. Prostate
34. Retina
35. Skin
36. Stomach
37. Testis
38. Thymus
39. Thyroid
40. Uterus
41. Yolk sac

table 2.2.1

In addition, scientists who have mapped the points at which vitamin D interacts with our DNA, have identified **over two thousand and a half genes.** The interaction of active vitamin D with these genes produces specific proteins with positive activities and functions. Some regulate calcium and phosphorus metabolism, whereas others act as sentinels of the body by preventing uncontrolled growth and then cancers, regulating insulin secretion in the pancreas, promoting serotonin production in the brain, affect the immune system.

Although most people think of vitamin D as just a vitamin, they often overlook the significant ways that it affects your bone, heart, brain, lung, liver, kidney, pancreas, immune system, inflammation system, and overall health. Here are some key roles of vitamin D:

Prevents and helps treat some types of cancers such as colon, breast, ovarian, and prostate cancers. Recent clinical and epidemiological studies have shown the role of Vitamin D in regulating cell growth, cell differentiation and proliferation, and cell death suggesting vitamin D exerts preventive actions in the instigation of cancer by interrupting the formation of cancer cells. Vitamin D may have beneficial effects in preventing the development of certain cancers and lowering their incidence, particularly when the total vitamin D [25(OH)D] level is more than **50 nanograms/mL (125 nmol/L).**

Prevents and helps treat cardiovascular diseases. Published studies have identified vitamin D as one of the most important factors in cardiovascular health due to its effects on various tissues and organs that participate in atherosclerosis and its regulatory effects in this systemic inflammatory process.
In contrast, vitamin D deficiency is associated with heart failure, heart attacks, strokes, peripheral arterial disease, and high blood pressure. Vitamin D exerts beneficial effects in preventing and reducing the incidence of cardiovascular diseases, particularly when the total vitamin D [25(OH)D] level is more than 40 nanograms/mL.

Prevents and helps treat type 1 diabetes, and type 2 diabetes. Vitamin D appears to play important role in regulating insulin secretion and in promoting the survival and health of pancreatic beta-cell responsible for making and secreting insulin. Thus, It is established that Vitamin D is essential for normal glucose metabolism and improvement of insulin sensitivity. Vitamin D has beneficial effects in preventing and lowering the severity of type 1 and type 2 diabetes, as well as gestational diabetes particularly when the total vitamin D [25(OH)D] level is more than 40 nanograms/mL.

Prevents and helps treat infections and disorders of the immune system. Recent studies and epidemiological data have indicated that vitamin D deficiency is positively correlated with the exacerbation of inflammatory autoimmune diseases and infectious diseases, such as rheumatoid arthritis, flu, and multiple sclerosis. Vitamin D directly affects immune cells and prevents the immune system from attacking the body's healthy cells. Vitamin D has beneficial effects in preventing and lowering the incidence and risks associated with infections and disorders of the immune system, particularly when the total vitamin D [25(OH)D] level is more than 40 nanograms/mL.

Prevents and helps treat bone disorders, falls, and fractures in the elderly. Vitamin D inadequacy is prevalent in the elderly due to various risk factors, including reduced sunlight exposure, deficient intestinal absorption, and impaired vitamin D activation in the liver and kidneys. Vitamin D inadequacy is prevalent in the elderly due to various risk factors, including reduced sunlight exposure, deficient intestinal absorption, and impaired vitamin D activation in the liver and kidneys. Vitamin D supplementation results in positive outcomes concerning fall prevention, particularly when patients reach and maintain a total vitamin D [25(OH)D] level of more than 40 nanograms/mL.

Prevents and helps treat reverse weight gain and obesity. It is suggested that the concentration of 25(OH)D is negatively correlated with the body mass index (BMI) and the percentage of fat mass. Vitamin D supplementation results in positive outcomes regarding weight gain and obesity, particularly when patients reach and maintain a total vitamin D [25(OH)D] level of more than 40 nanograms/mL.

Prevents and helps treat dementia, schizophrenia, and depression. Evidence from clinical studies has supported the association of vitamin D deficiency with many mental disorders, including schizophrenia and depression. Ongoing studies are conducted to bring more proof and support the potentially positive role of vitamin D in schizophrenia and depression treatments.

Prevents and helps treat pulmonary disease (including COPD and cystic fibrosis). Adequate vitamin D status has been recently associated with a significant decrease in the severity of some respiratory diseases such as Chronic obstructive pulmonary disease (COPD), tuberculosis, and cystic fibrosis).

Prevents and helps treat autoimmune diseases. Vitamin D exerts beneficial effects and produces good outcomes in the immune system due to its involvement in cellular development. Vitamin D directly affects immune cells and prevents the immune system from attacking the body's healthy cells. An adequate vitamin D status is associated with a reduced risk of developing autoimmune diseases such as type 1 diabetes, rheumatoid arthritis, thyrotoxicosis, Crohn's disease, psoriasis, ulcerative colitis, and polymyalgia. Vitamin D has beneficial effects in preventing and lowering the incidence and risks associated with infections and disorders of the immune system, particularly when the total vitamin D [25(OH)D] level is more than 40 nanograms/mL.

Prevents and helps treat parathyroid disorders. The association between vitamin D and the parathyroid hormone (PTH) was established by several studies due to its importance in bone remodeling in the elderly. Vitamin D-deficient patients were those who had higher values of PTH, while individuals with an adequate vitamin D status had low PTH values.

Prevents and helps treat allergies. Observational studies have established that vitamin D deficiency may contribute to the development and/or severity of asthma and allergic diseases. It is believed that a vitamin D [25(OH)D] level in the range of 40-60 nanograms/mL may be beneficial in the prevention of asthma and allergic diseases and the reduction of their incidence.

Prevents and helps treat rheumatoid arthritis. Vitamin D deficiency has been associated with the pathogenesis of autoimmune diseases, such as type I diabetes and rheumatoid arthritis.

Prevents and helps treat psoriasis. Vitamin D deficiency is linked to the development of autoimmune diseases such as psoriasis. Vitamin D has beneficial effects in preventing and lowering the incidence and risks associated with infections and disorders of the immune system, particularly when the total vitamin D [25(OH)D] level is more than 40 nanograms/mL.

Prevents and helps treat thyroid disorders. Current observational studies have suggested that deficiency of vitamin D and calcium levels were associated with the degree and severity of hypothyroidism. A vitamin D supplementation may alleviate symptoms and severity of thyroid disorders.

Prevents and helps treat cognitive decline. Recent studies have established that poor vitamin D levels are associated with a higher risk of cognitive decline.

Prevents and helps treat fibromyalgia. Vitamin D deficiency and insufficiency have been associated with fibromyalgia. The vitamin D [25(OH)D] levels in the range of 40-60 ng/ml seem to improve disease symptoms in patients with fibromyalgia.

Prevents and helps treat vision disorders. A growing body of evidence points to the association between vision disorders and vitamin D deficiency.

Prevents and helps treat autism spectrum disorders. Vitamin D may have beneficial outcomes in autism spectrum disorders subjects, particularly when the total vitamin D [25(OH)D] level is more than 40 nanograms/mL.

11

VITAMIN D REQUIREMENTS - THE BIG MISTAKE

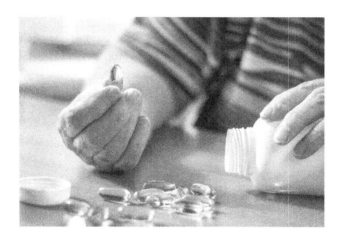

The amount of vitamin D needed per day is different for each person and corresponds to the adequate level of the vitamin D [25(OH)D] in the body to prevent all of the problems associated with vitamin D3 deficiency (bone pain, muscle weakness, increased autoimmunity, anxiety, depression, weight gain). However, A big calculation error has biased the vitamin D recommendations (RDAs) by the National Academy of Medicine. RDAs are far too low, by roughly a factor of ten.

————

There is strong evidence that increasing dietary vitamin D intake will safely lead to an increase in circulating 25(OH)D and thus improve people's vitamin D status. In the United States and Canada, in 2010, the National Academy of Medicine (NAM) —formerly called the Institute of Medicine— set the Recommended dietary allowance (RDA) to 600 IU (15 mcg) for everyone age 1–70 years, and the RDA of 800 IU (20 mcg) for adults over 70 years, and an adequate intake value of 400 IU (10 mcg) for infants below one year. The European Food Safety Authority set the same Similar RDAs values in 2016.

However, a growing body of evidence has pointed to these recommendations as undervalued and miscalculated. A multitude of observational studies has demonstrated that the current nutritional guidelines issued by the NAM and adopted in the United States, Canada, and Europe are far below the adequate level of daily vitamin D intake that will allow individuals to benefit from its many health properties.

The public health and clinical consequences of the published and underestimated vitamin D's RDAs are serious. People who rely on these recommendations and get 600 IU per day will never achieve vitamin D sufficiency and will experience poor outcomes of vitamin D deficiency, such as an increased risk of developing chronic inflammatory diseases, cancers, bone disorders[1], and cardiovascular diseases.

————

How much vitamin D should you take?

Checking out the United States government's recommendations

The expert panel of the Food and Nutrition Board at the National Academies of Sciences, Engineering, and Medicine has established recommended dietary allowances (RDAs) for vitamin D to indicate daily vitamin D intakes sufficient to prevent rickets and osteomalacia in healthy people —"normal calcium metabolism" and "bone health"— and that's all.

At the request of the United States and Canadian governments, the National Academy of Medicine (NAM) issues dietary recommendations, including the Recommended Dictary Allowance (RDA). The RDA is the average daily nutrient intake level considered sufficient to meet the requirements of 97.5 percent of healthy individuals.

In November 2010, the National Academy of Medicine significantly increased RDAs for all age groups: For individuals from 1 to 50 years old, the RDA increased from 200 to 600 international units (IU) a day; for individuals 50 to 70 years old, from 400 to 600 IU; and for people over 70, from 600 to 800 IU. The new RDAs were supposed to achieve circulating serum vitamin D [25(OH)D] levels of 20 nanograms/mL (50 nmol/L) in 97.5% of healthy individuals.

The dietary reference Allowances (RDAs) were founded upon data exploring the beneficial effects of vitamin D and calcium on skeletal and not extraskeletal health.

Following the vitamin D nonskeletal benefits perspective, the Endocrine Society decided to adopt 30 nanograms/mL (75 nmol/L) as the cut-off value of vitamin D sufficiency. And thus, people need substantially more vitamin D than the RDAs on the order of 1,500–2,000 IU per day to experience improvement in their overall health and well-being.

As you'll see, published Recommended dietary allowances (RDAs) for vitamin D are underestimated and miscalculated. The table below is only for further reference and is not intended for use. Most people need a much higher dose, estimated in a 2014 study to be 8992 IU for adults, and in a 2015 study to 7000 IU. In my perspective, and based on my experience and data analysis, In healthy *people*, the amount of vitamin D needed per day varies and depends on several factors, as you will see later in this chapter.

Age	Male	Female	Pregnancy	Lactation
0-12 months	10 mcg (400 IU)	10 mcg (400 IU)		
1–13 years	15 mcg (600 IU)	15 mcg (600 IU)		
14–18 years	15 mcg (600 IU)	15 mcg (600 IU)	15 mcg (600 IU)	15 mcg (600 IU)
19–50 years	15 mcg (600 IU)	15 mcg (600 IU)	15 mcg (600 IU)	15 mcg (600 IU)
51–70 years	15 mcg (600 IU)	15 mcg (600 IU)		
>70 years	20 mcg (800 IU)	20 mcg (800 IU)		

RDA for vitamin D underestimated by an order of magnitude

The public health and clinical implications of the published and miscalculated RDAs for vitamin D are serious. With the currently published recommendation of 600 IU, bone health objectives and chronic disease prevention goals will never be met. Because the correctly calculated RDAs, which corresponds to the correct daily vitamin D intake level considered as sufficient to meet the requirements of 97.5 percent of healthy individuals is more than 11 times higher.

Irrelevant recommendations of the RDAs based on outdated docu-

mentation. The NAM's Experts have updated these dietary allowances (RDAs) for vitamin D to indicate the optimal daily vitamin D intake enough to maintain "normal calcium metabolism" and "bone health" in healthy people.

Suppose you look at the statement above carefully. In that case, you will find that the expert panel of the Food and Nutrition Board established the RDAs for vitamin D to prevent rickets and osteomalacia in healthy people —*"normal calcium metabolism"* and *"bone health"*— and that's all.

In addition, we have to stress that these recommendations were mainly based on outdated published literature earlier than the 1980s when vitamin D was intended only to prevent rickets in children.

Today, there is a general agreement that children and adults need a minimum of 2,000 IU (50 mcg) of vitamin D per day to maintain a blood level of 25(OH)D above 30 nanograms per milliliter, promoting overall health.

The Big Mistake in the Estimation of RDAs. In a 2014 study, investigators Veugelers and Ekwaru have shown that the current RDAs were underestimated. The two scientists have established that the National Academy of Medicine made a Big statistical error that led to erroneous RDAs for Vitamin D.

Using the data of the National Academy of Medicine, they found that 8895 IU per day was needed for 97.5% of individuals to achieve values ≥20 nanograms/mL (50 nmol/L). Therefore, the correctly calculated RDA for vitamin D is 8895 IU per day (instead of 600 IU the published IOM RDAs) for individuals aged 1 to 70 years.

Another study published in 2015 confirmed that 6201 IU/d was needed to achieve 30 nanograms/mL (75 nmol/L), and 9122 IU/day was needed to reach (40 nanograms/mL) 100 nmol/L. Robert Heaney and Carole Baggerly have also established that the National Academy of Medicine made a big mistake in calculating vitamin D daily intake. They demonstrated that the total intake required to achieve 20 nanograms/mL (50 nmol/L) in 97.5% of individuals must be close to 7000 IU per day, not substantially different from the correctly calculated RDA in 2014.

In 2017, a study conducted by GrassrootsHealth concluded that 7,000 IU/day of vitamin D is needed to get 97.5% of the population to a minimum 20 ng/ml (50 nmol/L) level of vitamin D [25(OH)D] established by the National Academy of Medicine. To reach a serum level of 40-60 nanograms/mL recommended by the Endocrine Society to prevent skeletal and non-skeletal diseases, GrassrootsHealth established **that a daily intake of 12,000 IU from all source inputs is needed to get 97.5% of the population to 40 nanograms/mL (100 nmol/L).**

Public health and clinical implications of the Miscalculated RDA

The public health and clinical implications of the current RDAs for vitamin D are serious. Because the correctly calculated RDAs, which correspond to the correct daily vitamin D intake level considered sufficient to meet the requirements of 97.5 percent of healthy individuals, are more than 11 times higher.

As many doctors begin to apply what they learned about vitamin D correction, they find that many patients feel better after starting supplements with 50,000 IU megadose per week for six to eight weeks. They no longer suffer from muscle spasms, bone pain, joint pain, or high blood pressure. But, when patients get the recommended maintenance dose of 800-1,000 IU/day from dietary and supplemental sources, their vitamin D [25(OH)D] levels drop, and the beneficial health effects vanish.

Many clinical studies felt to show to beneficial effects of vitamin D in many diseases because they rely on the government's RDAs. They largely failed to show the significant effects of 600 IU vitamin D supplementation on various health outcomes. In contrast, in clinical studies based on high vitamin D supplementation, the beneficial vitamin D effects have been established on multiple health outcomes such as respiratory diseases, cancers, chronic inflammatory disorders, pregnancy outcomes, and mortality.

Tolerable Upper Intake Levels of vitamin D

In the last decade, from the United States to Europe, experts on Nutrition were asked to reevaluate the safety of vitamin D use and provide, if applicable, revised vitamin D (ULs) for relevant population groups.

The UL was established to 100 µg/day (4.000 IU/day) for ages 11-17 years. For children aged 1-10 years, the UL was adapted to 50 µg/day (2.000 IU/day), considering their smaller body size. The UL was set to 25 µg/day for infants under one year (1.000 IU/day).

Age	Male	Female	Pregnancy	Lactation
0-12 months	25 mcg (1000 IU)	25 mcg (1000 IU)		
1–10 years	50 mcg (2000 IU)	50 mcg (2000 IU)		
11–17 years	100 mcg (4000 IU)	100 mcg (4000 IU)	100 mcg (4000 IU)	100 mcg (4000 IU)
18–50 years	100 mcg (4000 IU)	100 mcg (4000 IU)	100 mcg (4000 IU)	100 mcg (4000 IU)
51–70 years	100 mcg (4000 IU)	100 mcg (4000 IU)		
>70 years	100 mcg (4000 IU)	100 mcg (4000 IU)		

A growing number of experts worldwide agree today that both children and adults need a minimum of 2,000 IU (50 mcg) of vitamin D per day to maintain a blood level of vitamin D [25(OH)D] above 30 nanograms per milliliter, considered as promoting overall health.

The vitamin D body's need is different for each person

It would be best to think of vitamin D as a hormone at this step. Would you then take mega-doses without knowing more about vitamin D toxicity?

In the chapters "Vitamin D Toxicity," and "Vitamin D Optimal Doses," you'll learn more about the adverse effects of extra-high doses of vitamin D, and more importantly, you'll be able to know your optimal dose of vitamin D3.

> Vitamin D deficiency is exacerbated during the winter season, and its incidence is higher among women than in men, higher in the elderly population than young ones, higher in obese people than nonobese ones, and higher among dark-skinned people than white ones.

The amount of vitamin D needed per day is different for each person and corresponds to the adequate level of the vitamin D [25(OH)D] in the body to prevent all of the problems associated with vitamin D3 deficiency (bone pain, muscle weakness, increased autoimmunity, anxiety, depression, weight gain). Thus, the amount of vitamin D [25(OH)D3] in your blood is a good indicator of how much vitamin D your body already has and how much it needs.

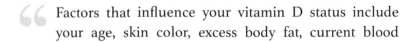 Factors that influence your vitamin D status include your age, skin color, excess body fat, current blood

vitamin D levels, Latitude of residence, lifestyle (sun exposure), and more.

Age and vitamin D requirements

Studies found that aging decreases significantly the cutaneous production of vitamin D3 by greater than twofold. Compared with younger, the elderly have lower levels of the 7-dehydrocholesterol in the skin that UVB light converts into the previtamin D3. According to a 2006 study, more than fifty percent of women and men aged 65 and older in North America are vitamin D–deficient.

People aged 65 years and older should take vitamin D3 supplementation to ensure they get the sufficient amount of vitamin D3 needed for bone and muscle health. As said earlier, vitamin D3 dose is different for each person. The Endocrine Society recommended for at-risk groups like those suffering from bone disease, kidney diseases, or liver malabsorption to take:

- 15–25 mcg per day (600–1000 IU) for children
- 37.5–50 mcg per day (1500–2000 IU) for adults

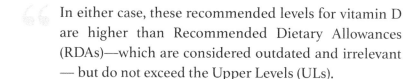

> In either case, these recommended levels for vitamin D are higher than Recommended Dietary Allowances (RDAs)—which are considered outdated and irrelevant — but do not exceed the Upper Levels (ULs).

Calculating optimal sun-exposure

Ola Engelsen, a scientist in the Department of Atmosphere and Climate at the Norwegian Institute for Air Research, has developed an online application to allow you to calculate the time you need in the sun to get a healthy dose of vitamin D3 without the risk of sunburn.

The calculator is available at this address:

(https://fastrt.nilu.no/VitD_quartMEDandMED_v2.html)

This calculator allows you to enter all the factors influencing your UVB exposure.

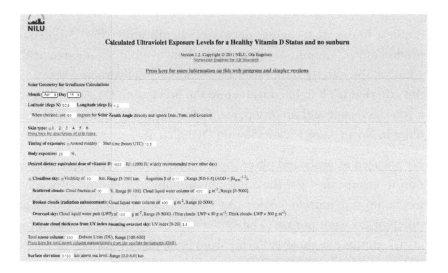

- These factors include:
- Desired dietary equivalent dose of vitamin D
- Residence Latitude
- Day and season of the year
- Skin type
- Body exposure
- Skin type
- Ground surface type

Limitations of this calculator:

Remember when using this calculator that even though it has undergone internal checking and validation, the model used is based only on one category of factors, those affecting the solar-ultraviolet B radiation such as latitude, altitude, time, clouds, aerosols, total ozone, and surface reflectivity.

Aging, for example, is recognized to decrease the capacity of human skin significantly to form vitamin D3.

---

1. **bone disorders** refer to medical conditions that damage the skeleton and make bones weak and susceptible to fractures. Some common bone diseases are osteoporosis, osteoarthritis, rickets, osteomalacia.

12

VITAMIN D STATUS FOR OPTIMAL HEALTH BENEFITS

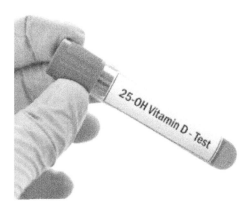

" Vitamin D status has been extensively studied in most countries of the world. The best determinant of vitamin D status is the serum concentration of 25-hydroxyvitamin D [25(OH)D]. There is no consensus on what constitutes optimal vitamin D blood levels. Some studies recommend 30 nanograms/mL (75 nmol/L), whereas others propose 40 to 60 nanograms/mL (100—150 nmol/L).

There is a huge and growing body of scientific literature and clinical studies for vitamin D deficiency. PUBMED (National Library of Medicine) lists ≥ 35,973 publications that use the keyword "**vitamin D status**" in either the title or abstract from 1945 to the present. This total includes articles that combine the use of **vitamin D deficiency** with one of the following terms:

- health (≥ 9,090 publications),
- adults (≥ 7,954 publications),
- children (≥ 3,744 publications),
- supplement (≥ 3,299 publications),
- diabetes (≥ 1,891 publications),
- cancer (≥ 1,779 publications),
- osteoporosis (≥ 1,584 publications),
- cardiovascular (≥ 1,288 publications),
- obesity (≥ 1,479 publications),
- chronic diseases (≥ 1,256 publications),
- infections (≥ 1,233 publications),
- immune (≥ 1,147 publications),
- inflammatory (≥ 983 publications).

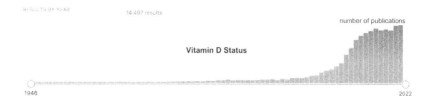

Finally, PUBMED lists ≥ 3,655 publications with the term vitamin D3 in the title or abstract, ≥ 710 articles with vitamin D2, and ≥ 1,303 articles with calcitriol [hormonally active vitamin D].

A circulating vitamin D [25(OH)D] level below 20 nanograms/L (50 nmol/L) is considered the lower threshold of vitamin D status and an indicator of vitamin D deficiency by the National Academy of Medicine (formerly IOM). However, this cut-off value was set only to prevent rickets in children and osteomalacia in adults.

Today, there is a growing acceptance of a much higher value of 30 nanograms/mL (75nmol/L) as the lower limit of the "sufficiency" range. The Endocrine Society suggested blood levels of circulating vitamin D [25(OH)D] at the range of 50 and 80 nanograms/mL (125 to 200 nmol/L) as optimal. More recently, the cut-off value for cancer prevention was set to 50 nanograms/nL.

Vitamin D Status: Measurement, Interpretation

Vitamin D produced in the skin or acquired in the diet is biologically inert and requires two-step-process hydroxylation first in the liver to form calcidiol (vitamin D metabolite [25(OH)D]), and then in the kidney plus many other body tissues to form calcitriol (vitamin D metabolite [1,25(OH)2D]).

Calcitriol is tightly regulated at the tissue level and is present in circulation only in the very lowest amounts; thus, the total vitamin D [25(OH)D] level is considered the more relevant blood circulating metabolite for assessing overall vitamin D status.

In 2010 the National Academy of Medicine issued a report based on a thorough examination of available data by a group of experts. They established that vitamin D level in the range of 30-50 nmol/L or 12-20 nanograms/ml is considered inadequate for bone health and overall health in healthy individuals and thus corresponds to vitamin D deficiency. (table 2)

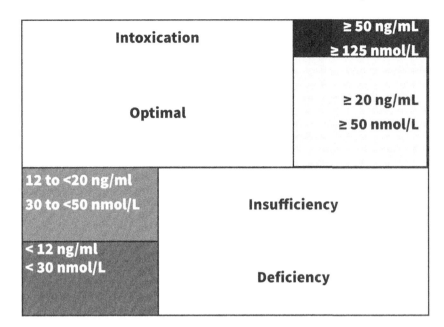

table 2. National Academy of Medicine Reference Ranges for total Serum 25-hydroxyvitamin D [25(OH)D]

However, the work of the National Academy of Medicine was based on outdated documentation and ignored many of the ongoing studies about the skeletal and non-skeletal functions of vitamin D. In 2011, the Endocrine Society took a more global perspective. It recommended adopting a much higher minimum blood level of 25(OH)D at 30 nanograms/mL (75nmol/L) for both children and adults. They also suggested that this would require 1500– 2000IU/day to achieve rather than 600 IU issued by the National Academy of Medicine. Based on a solid body of evidence, the Endocrine Society committee defined the optimal serum level of 25(OH)D between 40 and 60 nanograms/mL (100—150 nmol/L) for both children and adults.

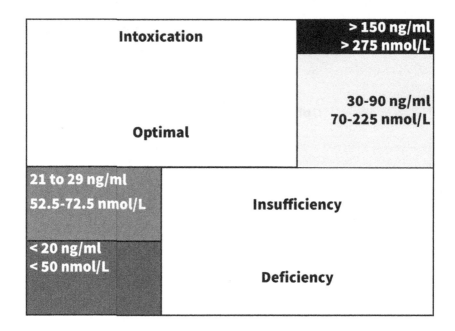

table 3. The Endocrine Society Reference Ranges for Total Serum 25-hydroxyvitamin D [25(OH)D]

- vitamin D deficiency occurs when the level of 25(OH)D in circulating human blood is less than or equal to 20 nanograms/ml (50 nmol/L),
- insufficiency occurs when the 25(OH)D level is between 21 to 29 nanograms/ml (52.5 to 72.5 nmol/L)
- sufficiency occurs if the 25(OH)D level is greater than or equal to 30 nanograms/ml. **The optimal zone to take full benefits of vitamin D is defined by 25(OH)D levels between 40 to 60 nanograms/ml (100 to 150 nmol/L)**
- toxic level of 25(OH)D above 150 nanograms/ml (275 nmol/L)

Poor vitamin D status impairs or damages many of the protective and reparative activities of vitamin D.

When should you get the vitamin D test?

The vitamin D blood level test may be requested for several reasons.

The blood test is the only accurate way to help doctors check and monitor your vitamin D status if you are at increased risk of having a vitamin D deficiency.

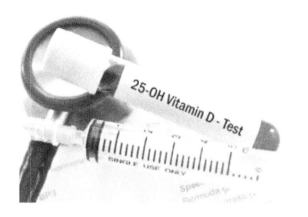

Most experts agree we should check vitamin D levels routinely in high-risk people. These include:

- dark-skinned people
- obese people (BMI greater than or equal to 30 kg/m2)
- people with skeletal disorders (e.g., osteoporosis, osteomalacia, osteopenia)
- people with gastrointestinal disorders (e.g., inflammatory bowel disease)
- people with anorexia nervosa
- people who had gastric bypass surgeries
- people with chronic kidney disease
- chronic liver diseases
- people with celiac disease or sprue
- people with endocrine disorders
- pregnant and lactating women

If your doctor asks you for a vitamin D test, ask more about your health risks, before getting the test. Your doctor may suspect a low vitamin D level. If this is the case taking a Vitamin D3 supplement may be sufficient.

13

VITAMIN D OPTIMAL DOSES

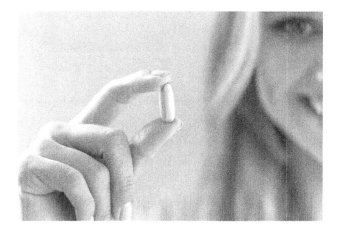

The circulating vitamin D [25(OH)D] concentration optimal to meet the physiological needs and produce positive outcomes of adults is a continuing subject of debate. Current recommendations show no consensus concerning the optimal vitamin D status, with conflicting recommendations defining serum 25(OH)D levels of 50 nanograms/mL as adequate and others advocating serum 25(OH)D levels in the range of 40-60 nanograms/mL. **We suggest blood levels of vitamin D [25(OH)D] in the range of 50 and 80 nanograms/mL (125 to 200 nmol/L),** which corresponds to the preventive cancer range.

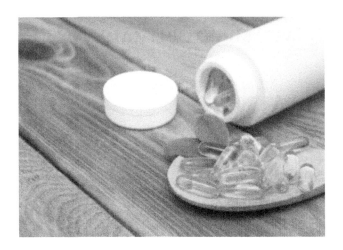

There is an emerging and growing body of scientific literature and clinical studies on the subject of "vitamin D high doses." PUBMED (National Library of Medicine) lists ≥ 2,863 publications that use the keyword "**vitamin D high doses**" in either the title or abstract from 1946 to the present. This total includes articles that combine the use of **vitamin D in high doses** with one of the following terms:

- health (≥ 900 publications),
- supplement (≥ 857 publications),
- kidney (≥ 427 publications),
- cancer (≥ 419 publications),
- chronic diseases (≥ 348 publications),
- osteoporosis (≥ 330 publications),
- diabetes (≥ 289 publications),
- safety (≥ 250 publications),
- inflammatory (≥ 241 publications),

- safety (≥ 240 publications),
- cardiovascular (≥ 240 publications),
- infections (≥ 213 publications),
- immune (≥ 185 publications),
- skin (≥ 151 publications),
- obesity (≥ 105 publications).

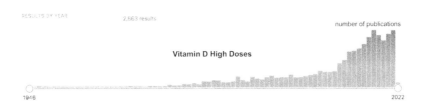

Finally, PUBMED lists ≥ 1,732 publications with the term vitamin D3 in the title or abstract, ≥ 221 articles with vitamin D2, and ≥ 756 articles with calcitriol [hormonally active vitamin D].

There is an emerging consensus that if you achieve adequate vitamin D status, you will experience many beneficial health outcomes covering a wide range of skeletal, cardiovascular, malignant, autoimmune, metabolic, infectious, and other conditions. This include:

- certain types of cancers such as colon, breast, ovarian, and prostate cancers.
- cardiovascular diseases.
- type 1 diabetes, type 2 diabetes.
- infections and disorders of the immune system.
- falls in the elderly.
- weight gain and obesity.
- dementia, schizophrenia and depression.
- autoimmune diseases
- acne

- allergies
- arthritis
- cognitive decline
- multiple sclerosis
- memory loss
- vision disorders
- autism spectrum disorders
- asthma and breathing disorders
- chronic fatigue
- chronic pain
- cystic fibrosis
- fibromyalgia
- migraines
- psoriasis
- thyroid disorders
- parathyroid disorders

On the basis of the available evidence, optimal dosing of vitamin D3 will improve your life, help reverse some chronic diseases, and prevent many medical conditions. By taking the optimal level of vitamin D3—with the right amounts of magnesium and vitamin K2 —you will safely experience the many health benefits that come with it.

Optimal dosing of vitamin D3 is safe, effective, and works. I personally take supplementation of 7,000 IU of vitamin D3 a day, with 500 mg of magnesium and 200 mcg of vitamin K2 (MK-7).

The safety of optimal dosing is based upon available evidence that has established the following facts.

- In healthy individuals, no adverse outcomes were reported giving 11,000 IU per day for five months.
- A daily intake of 10,000 IU of vitamin D over prolonged

periods did not cause toxicity, even when individuals received significant solar-UVB exposure to bare skin.

- The vitamin D administration at 1000 mcg (40,000 IU) per day induces toxic effects in the infant within 1 to 4 months. In adults, administration of 1250 mcg (50,000 IU) per day for several months can lead, in rare cases, to intoxication.

In 2017, a study conducted by GrassrootsHealth concluded that 7,000 IU/day of vitamin D is needed to get 97.5% of the population to a minimum of 20 nanograms/ml (50 nmol/L) of circulating vitamin D [25(OH)D] established by the National Academy of Medicine. In addition, to reach a serum level of 40-60 nanograms/mL, which the Endocrine Society recommends to prevent skeletal and non-skeletal diseases, GrassrootsHealth established **that a daily intake of 12,000 IU from all source inputs is needed to get 97.5% of the population to 40 nanograms/mL (100 nmol/L).**

Vitamin D correction — The Optimal Doses

Your starting point is to check your vitamin D [25(OH)D] level in the blood and refer to the next paragraph to identify your vitamin D status.

The optimal vitamin D [25(OH)D] level is between 50 and 80 nanograms/mL (125 to 200 nmol/L), which corresponds to the preventive cancer range based on strong evidence about the association between vitamin D and beneficial health outcomes, including cancer prevention, and treatment of some conditions including Psoriatic arthritis, asthma, rheumatoid arthritis, and tuberculosis.

Or between 40 and 60 nanograms/mL (125 to 200 nmol/L) as the Endocrine Society recommends based on strong and growing evidence about the association between vitamin D and many conditions, including bone disorders (rickets in children, osteomalacia in adults, and osteoporosis), diabetes, multiple sclerosis, rheumatoid arthritis, cancer, and many others.

Vitamin D status and its management for achieving optimal health benefits

You'll then be able to identify your vitamin D status and determine the optimal dosing for you by referring to the relevant paragraph:

- If your vitamin D level is below 20 nanograms/mL (50 nmol/L), then refer to paragraph (I)
- If your vitamin D level is in the range of 21-29 nanograms/mL (52.5-72.5 nmol/L), then refer to paragraph (II)
- If your vitamin D level is in the range of 30-90 nanograms/mL (70-225 nmol/L), then refer to paragraph (III)
- If your vitamin D level is higher than 110 nanograms/mL (275 nmol/L), then refer to paragraph (IV)

I. You have severe vitamin D deficiency

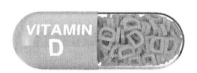

It corresponds to your total serum vitamin D [25(OH)D] concentration. It is obtained by a vitamin D blood test.

The vitamin D blood test measures the concentration of the vitamin D metabolite calcidiol ([25(OH)D]) in your blood.

The vitamin D blood test measures the concentration of the vitamin D metabolite calcidiol ([25(OH)D]) in your blood.

If your blood results show a low vitamin D level, it may indicate you are:

- not getting sufficient exposure to sunlight
- not taking adequate vitamin D in your diet
- having some disorders that alter vitamin D absorption in the intestines
- having some factors that lower the production of vitamin D in the skin (age above 65, obesity, dark skin)

In the United States and several other countries, levels are measured using nanograms per milliliter or nanograms/mL. To convert nanograms/mL to nmol/L, just **multiply the nanograms/mL by 2.5.** For example, 40 nanograms/mL is equivalent to 100 nmol/L.

I.2. Your desired Serum Level

It corresponds to the value you aim to achieve in the range of 50-80 nanograms/mL, which corresponds to the preventive range of cancer. You can also choose the optimal range recommended by the Endocrine Society between 40 to 60 nanograms/mL.

The difference between your desired serum level and your starting vitamin D level corresponds to the desired rise in vitamin D level.

I.3. Your loading Dose

The loading dose of vitamin D3 is the amount of vitamin D3 needed to rapidly correct serum vitamin D [25(OH)D] level. The calculation of the loading dose is based on the works of van Groningen et al. in 2010. It depends on the degree of vitamin D deficiency, the desired rise in vitamin D level, and body weight as follows:

Vitamin D3 Loading dose (IU) = 47.5 multiplied by [target vitamin D level – starting vitamin D level (in nmol/L)] multiplied by body weight in kg.

This formula was adjusted for all adults regardless of their weight status (non-obese and obese people). Loading is typically oral and persists in the body for 1 to 3 months. The loading dose must be followed up with ongoing maintenance dosing.

Example 1:

- Subject: female, non-pregnant, and non-lactating
- Weight: 65 kg
- Starting vitamin D level: 15 nanograms/mL (37.5 nmol/L)
- Target vitamin D level: 50 nanograms/mL (125 nmol/L)
- Vitamin D3 Loading dose (IU) = 47.5 multiplied by (125 – 37.5) multiplied by 65
- Vitamin D3 Loading dose (IU)= 270,156 IU
- Ideally, the loading dose to correct vitamin D may be taken in 4 weeks. So, you have to divide by 4 the Vitamin D3 Loading dose (IU)= 270,156 IU, and you'll obtain 67,500 per week, approximately 10.000 IU per day for 28 days. (Loading doses can be taken as a single dose or slowly as two months.)

Example 2:

- Subject: female, non-pregnant and non-lactating
- Weight: 77 kg
- Starting vitamin D level: 15 nanograms/mL (37.5 nmol/L)
- Target vitamin D level: 50 nanograms/mL (125 nmol/L)
- Vitamin D3 Loading dose (IU) = 47.5 multiplied by (125 – 37.5) multiplied by 77
- Vitamin D3 Loading dose (IU)= 320,031 IU
- Ideally, the loading dose to correct vitamin D should be taken in 4 weeks. So, you have to divide by 4 the Vitamin D3 Loading dose (IU)= 320,031 IU, and you'll obtain roughly

80,000 per week, approximately 11.500 IU per day for 28 days. (Loading doses can be taken as a single dose or slowly as two months.)

I.4. The Maintenance Dose

The maintenance dose corresponds to the estimated amount of vitamin D3 intake needed to sustain the desired serum vitamin D [25(OH)D] concentration—in addition to all other natural inputs (food and the sun). The maintenance dose is intended to gradually increase your vitamin D levels to reach the desired target over approximately three months.

The calculation of the maintenance dose depends on the body weight of non-obese persons as follows:

Vitamin D3 Maintenance dose (IU) = 90 multiplied by body weight in kg.

For obese individuals and people with medical conditions affecting the absorption of vitamin D, the maintenance dose should be increased by 25%. Subjects are advised to consult with their physicians or other healthcare providers.

Here are some examples of daily maintenance doses:

- 50 kg: 4,500 IU
- 55 kg: 4,950 IU
- 60 kg: 5,400 IU
- 65 kg: 5,850 IU
- 70 kg: 6,300 IU
- 75 kg: 6,750 IU
- 80 kg: 7,200 IU
- 85 kg: 7,650 IU
- 90 kg: 8,100 IU

- 95 kg: 8,550 IU
- 100 kg: 9,000 IU
- 105 kg: 9,450 IU
- 110 kg: 9,900 IU

The calculated daily vitamin D intake for a 110 kg subject is 9900 IU under the 10,000 IU per day corresponding to No Observed Adverse Effect Level (NOAEL).

If you have the correct absorptive capacity, you'll expect to see your vitamin D [25(OH)D] concentrations increase by roughly 0.15—0.3 nanograms/mL (0.375—0.75 nmol/L) for every 50 IU/day (1 mcg/day) of vitamin D3 you take depending on your body weight.

Example 1:

- Subject: female, non-pregnant and non-lactating
- weight: 77 kg,
- The subject has a correct absorptive capacity,
- The subject has a BMI = 24.5 (normal)
- The calculated maintenance dose is: 6930 (roughly 7,000) IU daily intake
- This maintenance dose will allow the subject to keep her serum vitamin D [25(OH)D] higher than 40 nanograms/mL after a successful fill-up period.
- High doses of vitamin D3, up to 50,000 IU daily, may be necessary for patients with malabsorption conditions3. Subjects are advised to consult with their physicians or other healthcare providers.

Example 2:

- Subject: female, non-pregnant and non-lactating
- weight: 55 kg,
- The subject has a correct absorptive capacity,
- The subject has a BMI = 20.5 (normal)

- The calculated maintenance dose is: 4,950 (roughly 5,000) IU daily intake
- High doses of vitamin D3, up to 50,000 IU daily, may be necessary for patients with malabsorption conditions4. Subjects are advised to consult with their physicians or other healthcare providers.

Example 3:

- Subject: male
- weight: 140 kg,
- The subject has a correct absorptive capacity,
- The subject has a BMI = 32 (obese)
- The calculated maintenance dose is: 12,600 IU daily intake
- The adjusted maintenance dose is: 15,120 (roughly 15,000) IU daily intake
- The adjusted maintenance dose will allow the subject to raise his serum vitamin D [25(OH)D] after a successful fill-up period. However, due to the poor bioavailability of vitamin D in obese people, blood monitoring of vitamin D each three month may be necessary. Routine monitoring is necessary for patients that have malabsorption syndrome, obesity, or other conditions related to poor bioavailability of vitamin D.

I.5. Optimal Magnesium Dose

As all enzymes that metabolize vitamin D require magnesium, in addition to natural sources, supplementation of magnesium (300–600 mg/day) should be considered. Otherwise, you may see little to no improvement in your overall health when taking the optimal dose of vitamin D.

The amount of magnesium your body needs on a day-to-day basis is strongly dependent on your size and lifestyle. You can use this calculator to know approximately how much magnesium you should consume each day for optimal health outcomes.

https://www.biospherenutrition.co.nz/blogs/magnesium/how-much-magnesium-should-i-take

---

I.6. Vitamin K2 Optimal Doses

As for magnesium, most people need to increase the amount of vitamin k2 they typically consume. Table II.5.1 below is given as a reference so that you can estimate the amount of vitamin K2 daily intake.

- for **50 kg** body weight and **4,500 IU** daily vitamin D3 supplementation; the vitamin K2 supplementation is **200 mcg** daily
- for **55 kg** body weight and **4,950 IU** daily vitamin D3 supplementation; the vitamin K2 supplementation is **220 mcg** daily
- for **60 kg** body weight and **5,400 IU** daily vitamin D3 supplementation; the vitamin K2 supplementation is **240 mcg** daily
- for **65 kg** body weight and **5,850 IU** daily vitamin D3 supplementation; the vitamin K2 supplementation is **260 mcg** daily
- for **70 kg** body weight and **6,300 IU** daily vitamin D3 supplementation; the vitamin K2 supplementation is **280 mcg** daily
- for **75 kg** body weight and **6,750 IU** daily vitamin D3 supplementation; the vitamin K2 supplementation is **300 mcg** daily
- for **80 kg** body weight and **7,200 IU** daily vitamin D3

supplementation; the vitamin K2 supplementation is 320 mcg daily

- for **85 kg** body weight and **7,650 IU** daily vitamin D3 supplementation; the vitamin K2 supplementation is 340 mcg daily
- for **90 kg** body weight and **8,100 IU** daily vitamin D3 supplementation; the vitamin K2 supplementation is 360 mcg daily
- for **95 kg** body weight and **8,550 IU** daily vitamin D3 supplementation; the vitamin K2 supplementation is 380 mcg daily
- for **100 kg** body weight and **9,000 IU** daily vitamin D3 supplementation; the vitamin K2 supplementation is 400 mcg daily
- for **105 kg** body weight and **9,450 IU** daily vitamin D3 supplementation; the vitamin K2 supplementation is 420 mcg daily
- for **110 kg** body weight and **9,900 IU** daily vitamin D3 supplementation; the vitamin K2 supplementation is 440 mcg daily

table II.5.1

For values that are not in table II.5.1 you have to use the extrapolation formula:

The estimated vitamin K2 dose (mcg) = multiply the calculated maintenance dose by 4.5 and divide by 100

Example 1:

- Subject: female, non-pregnant and non-lactating
- weight: 77 kg,
- The subject has a correct absorptive capacity,
- The subject has a BMI = 24.5 (normal)

- The calculated maintenance dose is: 6930 (roughly 7,000) IU daily intake
- The estimated vitamin K2 dose is extrapolated to **310 mcg.** Because for 75 kg body weight and 6,750 IU daily vitamin D3 supplementation, the vitamin K2 supplementation is 300 mcg daily; and for 80 kg body weight and 7,200 IU daily vitamin D3 supplementation, the vitamin K2 supplementation is 320 mcg daily

Example 2:

- Subject: female, non-pregnant and non-lactating
- weight: 59 kg,
- The subject has a correct absorptive capacity,
- The subject has a BMI = 20.5 (normal)
- The calculated maintenance dose is: 5310 (roughly 5,300) IU daily intake
- The estimated vitamin K2 dose is extrapolated to **240 mcg.** Because of 60 kg body weight and 5,400 IU daily vitamin D3 supplementation.

Example 3:

- Subject: male
- weight: 140 kg,
- The subject has a correct absorptive capacity,
- The subject has a BMI = 32 (obese)
- The calculated maintenance dose is: 12,600 IU daily intake
- The adjusted maintenance dose is: 15,120 (roughly 15,000) IU daily intake
- The estimated vitamin K2 dose is extrapolated based on the calculated maintenance dose (12,600 IU) and not the adjusted maintenance dose. The estimated vitamin K2 dose is extrapolated to **560 mcg.**

I. 7. Additional factors to take into account

If you are taking medications that reduce the absorption of vitamin D, consider increasing your vitamin D intake by up to 20 percent. (see chapter "Factors Influencing Vitamin D Status")

If you are obese (body mass index (BMI) of 30) or have fat malabsorption syndrome, consider increasing your vitamin D intake by up to 20 percent.

To obtain the optimal vitamin D's beneficial effect on your bone health, you have to ingest, either from supplements or the diet, 1,000 milligrams of calcium a day if you are under fifty years and 1,200 milligrams of calcium if you are over fifty years.

Caution should be observed in patients with impairment of renal function, cardiovascular diseases, tuberculosis, or chronic fungal infections.

II. If you are vitamin D-insufficient

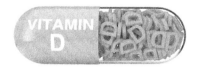

II.1. Your starting vitamin D level

It corresponds to your total serum vitamin D [25(OH)D] concentration. It is obtained by a vitamin D blood test.

The vitamin D blood test measures the concentration of the vitamin D metabolite calcidiol ([25(OH)D]) in your blood.

The vitamin D blood test measures the concentration of the vitamin D metabolite calcidiol ([25(OH)D]) in your blood.

If your blood results show a low vitamin D level, it may indicate you are:

- not getting sufficient exposure to sunlight
- not taking adequate vitamin D in your diet
- having some disorders that alter vitamin D absorption in the intestines
- having some factors that lower the production of vitamin D in the skin (age above 65, obesity, dark skin)

In the United States and several other countries, levels are measured using nanograms per milliliter or nanograms/mL. To convert nanograms/mL to nmol/L, just **multiply the nanograms/mL by 2.5.** For example, 40 nanograms/mL is equivalent to 100 nmol/L.

II.2. Your desired Serum Level

It corresponds to the value you aim to achieve in the range of 50-80 nanograms/mL, which corresponds to the preventive range of cancer. You can also choose the optimal range recommended by the Endocrine Society between 40 to 60 nanograms/mL.

The difference between your desired serum level and your starting vitamin D level corresponds to the desired rise in vitamin D level.

II.3. Your loading Dose

The loading dose of vitamin D3 is the amount of vitamin D3 needed to rapidly correct serum vitamin D [25(OH)D] level. The calculation of the loading dose is based on the works of van Groningen et al. in 2010. It depends on the degree of vitamin D deficiency, the desired rise in vitamin D level, and body weight as follows:

Vitamin D3 Loading dose (IU) = 40 multiplied by (target vitamin D level – starting vitamin D level (in nmol/L)) multiplied by body weight in kg.

This formula was adjusted for all adults regardless of their weight status (non-obese and obese people). Loading is typically oral and persists in the body for 1 to 3 months. The loading dose must be followed up with ongoing maintenance dosing.

Example 1:

- Subject: female, non-pregnant and non-lactating
- Weight: 65 kg
- Starting vitamin D level: 25 nanograms/mL (62.5 nmol/L)
- Target vitamin D level: 50 nanograms/mL (125 nmol/L)
- Vitamin D3 Loading dose (IU) = 40 multiplied by (125 – 62.5) multiplied by 65
- Vitamin D3 Loading dose (IU)= 162,500 IU
- Ideally, the loading dose to correct vitamin D insufficiency may be taken in 2 weeks. So, you have to divide by two the Vitamin D3 Loading dose (IU)= 162,500 IU, and you'll obtain 81,250 per week, approximately 11,600 IU per day for 14 days. (Loading doses can be taken as a single dose or slowly as two months.)

Example 2:

- Subject: female, non-pregnant, and non-lactating

- Weight: 77 kg
- Starting vitamin D level: 27 nanograms/mL (67.5 nmol/L)
- Target vitamin D level: 50 nanograms/mL (125 nmol/L)
- Vitamin D3 Loading dose (IU) = 40 multiplied by (125 – 37.5) multiplied by 77
- Vitamin D3 Loading dose (IU)= 177,100 IU (roughly 177,100 IU)
- Ideally, the loading dose to correct vitamin D insufficiency should be taken in 2 weeks. So, you have to divide by 4 the Vitamin D3 Loading dose (IU)= 270,000 IU, and you'll obtain roughly 88,500 per week, approximately 12.600 IU per day for 14 days. (Loading doses can be taken as a single dose or slowly as two months.)

II.4. The Maintenance Dose

The maintenance dose corresponds to the estimated amount of vitamin D3 intake needed to sustain the desired serum vitamin D [25(OH)D] concentration—in addition to all other natural inputs (food and the sun). The maintenance dose is intended to gradually increase vitamin D levels to reach the desired target over approximately three months.

The calculation of the maintenance dose depends on the body weight of non-obese persons as follows:

Vitamin D3 Maintenance dose (IU) = 90 multiplied by body weight in kg.

For obese individuals and people with medical conditions affecting the absorption of vitamin D, the maintenance dose should be increased by 25%. Subjects are advised to consult with their physicians or other healthcare providers.

Here are some examples of daily maintenance doses:

- 50 kg: 4,500 IU
- 55 kg: 4,950 IU
- 60 kg: 5,400 IU
- 65 kg: 5,850 IU
- 70 kg: 6,300 IU
- 75 kg: 6,750 IU
- 80 kg: 7,200 IU
- 85 kg: 7,650 IU
- 90 kg: 8,100 IU
- 95 kg: 8,550 IU
- 100 kg: 9,000 IU
- 105 kg: 9,450 IU
- 110 kg: 9,900 IU

The calculated daily vitamin D intake for a 110 kg subject is 9900 IU under the 10,000 IU per day corresponding to No Observed Adverse Effect Level (NOAEL).

If you have the correct absorptive capacity, you'll expect to see your vitamin D [25(OH)D] concentrations increase by roughly 0.15—0.3 nanograms/mL (0.375—0.75 nmol/L) for every 50 IU/day (1 mcg/day) of vitamin D3 you take depending on your body weight.

Example 1:

- Subject: female, non-pregnant and non-lactating
- weight: 77 kg,
- The subject has a correct absorptive capacity,
- The subject has a BMI = 24.5 (normal)
- The calculated maintenance dose is: 6930 (roughly 7,000) IU daily intake
- This maintenance dose may allow the subject to keep her serum vitamin D [25(OH)D] higher than 40 nanograms/mL after a successful loading.

High doses of vitamin D3, up to 50,000 IU daily, may be necessary for patients with malabsorption conditions5. Subjects are advised to consult with their physicians or other healthcare providers.

Example 2:

- Subject: female, non-pregnant and non-lactating
- weight: 55 kg,
- The subject has a correct absorptive capacity,
- The subject has a BMI = 20.5 (normal)
- The calculated maintenance dose is 4,950 (roughly 5,000) IU daily intake.
- This maintenance dose may allow the subject to keep her serum vitamin D [25(OH)D] higher than 40 nanograms/mL after a successful loading.

High doses of vitamin D3, up to 50,000 IU daily, may be necessary for patients with malabsorption conditions6. Subjects are advised to consult with their physicians or other healthcare providers.

Example 3:

- Subject: male
- weight: 140 kg,
- The subject has a correct absorptive capacity,
- The subject has a BMI = 32 (obese)
- The calculated maintenance dose is: 12,600 IU daily intake
- The adjusted maintenance dose is: 15,120 (roughly 15,000) IU daily intake (adjusted maintenance dose = calculated maintenance dose multiplied by 1.20)
- The adjusted maintenance dose will allow the subject to raise his serum vitamin D [25(OH)D] after a successful fill-up period. However, due to the poor bioavailability of vitamin D in obese people, blood monitoring of vitamin D each three month may be necessary.

II.5. Optimal Magnesium Dose

As all enzymes that metabolize vitamin D require magnesium, in addition to natural sources, supplementation of magnesium (300–600 mg/day) should be considered. Otherwise, you may see little to no improvement in your overall health when taking the optimal dose of vitamin D.

The amount of magnesium your body needs on a day-to-day basis is strongly dependent on your size and lifestyle. You can use this calculator to know approximately how much magnesium you should consume each day for optimal health outcomes.

https://www.biospherenutrition.co.nz/blogs/magnesium/how-much-magnesium-should-i-take

II.6. Vitamin K2 Optimal Doses

As for magnesium, most people need to increase the amount of vitamin k2 they typically consume. Table II.5.1 below is given as a reference so that you can estimate the amount of vitamin K2 daily intake.

- for **50 kg** body weight and **4,500 IU** daily vitamin D3 supplementation; the vitamin K2 supplementation is **200 mcg** daily
- for **55 kg** body weight and **4,950** IU daily vitamin D3 supplementation; the vitamin K2 supplementation is **220 mcg** daily
- for **60 kg** body weight and **5,400 IU** daily vitamin D3 supplementation; the vitamin K2 supplementation is **240 mcg** daily
- for **65 kg** body weight and **5,850 IU** daily vitamin D3 supplementation; the vitamin K2 supplementation is **260 mcg** daily

- for **70 kg** body weight and **6,300 IU** daily vitamin D3 supplementation; the vitamin K2 supplementation is **280 mcg** daily
- for **75 kg** body weight and **6,750 IU** daily vitamin D3 supplementation; the vitamin K2 supplementation is **300 mcg** daily
- for **80 kg** body weight and **7,200 IU** daily vitamin D3 supplementation; the vitamin K2 supplementation is **320 mcg** daily
- for **85 kg** body weight and **7,650 IU** daily vitamin D3 supplementation; the vitamin K2 supplementation is **340 mcg** daily
- for **90 kg** body weight and **8,100 IU** daily vitamin D3 supplementation; the vitamin K2 supplementation is **360 mcg** daily
- for **95 kg** body weight and **8,550 IU** daily vitamin D3 supplementation; the vitamin K2 supplementation is **380 mcg** daily
- for **100 kg** body weight and **9,000 IU** daily vitamin D3 supplementation; the vitamin K2 supplementation is **400 mcg** daily
- for **105 kg** body weight and **9,450 IU** daily vitamin D3 supplementation; the vitamin K2 supplementation is **420 mcg** daily
- for **110 kg** body weight and **9,900 IU** daily vitamin D3 supplementation; the vitamin K2 supplementation is **440 mcg** daily

table 2.5.1

For values that are not in the table, you have to use the extrapolation formula:

The estimated vitamin K2 dose (mcg) = multiply the calculated maintenance dose by 4.5 and divide by 100

Example 1:

- Subject: female, non-pregnant and non-lactating
- weight: 77 kg,
- The subject has a correct absorptive capacity,
- The subject has a BMI = 24.5 (normal)
- The calculated maintenance dose is: 6930 (roughly 7,000) IU daily intake
- The estimated vitamin K2 dose is extrapolated to **310 mcg.** Because for 75 kg body weight and 6,750 IU daily vitamin D3 supplementation, the vitamin K2 supplementation is 300 mcg daily; and for 80 kg body weight and 7,200 IU daily vitamin D3 supplementation, the vitamin K2 supplementation is 320 mcg daily

Example 2:

- Subject: female, non-pregnant and non-lactating
- weight: 59 kg,
- The subject has a correct absorptive capacity,
- The subject has a BMI = 20.5 (normal)
- The calculated maintenance dose is: 5310 (roughly 5,300) IU daily intake
- The estimated vitamin K2 dose is extrapolated to **240 mcg.** Because of 60 kg body weight and 5,400 IU daily vitamin D3 supplementation.

Example 3:

- Subject: male
- weight: 140 kg,
- The subject has a correct absorptive capacity,
- The subject has a BMI = 32 (obese)
- The calculated maintenance dose is: 12,600 IU daily intake

- The adjusted maintenance dose is: 15,120 (roughly 15,000) IU daily intake
- The estimated vitamin K2 dose is extrapolated based on the calculated maintenance dose (12,600 IU) and not the adjusted maintenance dose. The estimated vitamin K2 dose is extrapolated to **560 mcg.**

II.7. Additional factors to take into account

If you are taking medications that reduce the absorption of vitamin D, consider increasing your vitamin D intake by up to 20 percent. (see chapter "Factors Influencing Vitamin D Status")

If you are obese (body mass index (BMI) of 30) or have fat malabsorption syndrome, consider increasing your vitamin D intake by up to 20 percent.

To obtain the optimal vitamin D's beneficial effect on your bone health, you have to ingest, either from supplements or the diet, 1,000 milligrams of calcium a day if you are under fifty years and 1,200 milligrams of calcium if you are over fifty years.

Caution should be observed in patients with impairment of renal function, cardiovascular diseases, tuberculosis, or chronic fungal infections.

III. If you have an adequate vitamin D level

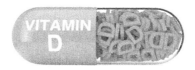

III.1. Your starting vitamin D level

It corresponds to your total serum vitamin D [25(OH)D] concentration. It is obtained by a vitamin D blood test.

The vitamin D blood test measures the concentration of the vitamin D metabolite calcidiol ([25(OH)D]) in your blood.

- **Suppose your vitamin D level is in the range of 30-50 nanograms/mL (75-100 nmol/L).** It would be best if you considered raising your vitamin D [25(OH)D] level to 50 nanograms/mL (125 nmol/L).
- **Suppose your vitamin D level is in the range of 50-90 nanograms/mL (125-225 nmol/L).** You already have an optimal vitamin D status and have to keep it by maintaining your lifestyle and nutritional habits. Therefore skip to the next chapter.

III.2. Your desired Serum Level

It corresponds to the value you aim to achieve in the range of 50-80 nanograms/mL, which corresponds to the preventive range of cancer. You can also choose the optimal range recommended by the Endocrine Society between 40 to 60 nanograms/mL.

The difference between your desired serum level and your starting vitamin D level corresponds to the desired rise in vitamin D level.

III.3. The Maintenance Dose

The maintenance dose corresponds to the estimated amount of vitamin D3 intake needed to sustain the desired serum vitamin D [25(OH)D] concentration—in addition to all other natural inputs (food and the sun). The maintenance dose is intended to gradually increase your vitamin D levels to reach the desired target over approximately three months.

The calculation of the maintenance dose depends on the body weight of non-obese persons as follows:

Vitamin D3 Maintenance dose (IU) = 90 multiplied by body weight in kg.

For obese individuals and people with medical conditions affecting the absorption of vitamin D, the maintenance dose should be increased by up to 20%. Subjects are advised to consult with their physicians or other healthcare providers.

Here are some examples of daily maintenance doses:

- 50 kg: 4,500 IU
- 55 kg: 4,950 IU
- 60 kg: 5,400 IU
- 65 kg: 5,850 IU
- 70 kg: 6,300 IU
- 75 kg: 6,750 IU
- 80 kg: 7,200 IU
- 85 kg: 7,650 IU
- 90 kg: 8,100 IU
- 95 kg: 8,550 IU
- 100 kg: 9,000 IU
- 105 kg: 9,450 IU
- 110 kg: 9,900 IU

The calculated daily vitamin D intake for a 110 kg subject is 9900 IU under the 10,000 IU per day corresponding to No Observed Adverse Effect Level (NOAEL).

If you have the correct absorptive capacity, you'll expect to see your vitamin D [25(OH)D] concentrations increase by roughly 0.15—0.3 nanograms/mL (0.375—0.75 nmol/L) for every 50 IU/day (1 mcg/day) of vitamin D3 you take depending on your body weight.

Example 1:

- Subject: female, non-pregnant and non-lactating
- weight: 48 kg,
- Subject has a correct absorptive capacity,
- The subject has a BMI = 21.5 (normal)
- The calculated maintenance dose is: 4,320 (roughly 4,300) IU daily intake
- This maintenance dose may allow the subject to keep her serum vitamin D [25(OH)D] higher than 40 nanograms/mL after a successful loading.

Example 2:

- Subject: female, non-pregnant and non-lactating
- weight: 69 kg,
- The subject has a correct absorptive capacity,
- The subject has a BMI = 22.5 (normal)
- The calculated maintenance dose is 6,210 (roughly 6,200) IU daily intake.
- This maintenance dose may allow the subject to keep her serum vitamin D [25(OH)D] higher than 40 nanograms/mL after a successful loading.

Example 3:

- Subject: female
- weight: 78 kg,

- The subject has a correct absorptive capacity,
- The subject has a BMI = 31 (obese)
- The calculated maintenance dose is: 7,020 IU daily intake
- The adjusted maintenance dose is: 8,424 (roughly 8,400) IU daily intake (adjusted maintenance dose = calculated maintenance dose multiplied by 1.20)
- The adjusted maintenance dose will allow the subject to raise his serum vitamin D [25(OH)D] after a successful fill-up period. However, due to the poor bioavailability of vitamin D in obese people, blood monitoring of vitamin D each three month may be necessary.

Magnesium Optimal Dose

As all enzymes that metabolize vitamin D require magnesium, in addition to natural sources, supplementation of magnesium (300–600 mg/day) should be considered. Otherwise, you may see little to no improvement in your overall health when taking the optimal dose of vitamin D.

The amount of magnesium your body needs on a day-to-day basis is strongly dependent on your size and lifestyle. You can use this calculator to know approximately how much magnesium you should consume each day for optimal health outcomes.

https://www.biospherenutrition.co.nz/blogs/magnesium/how-much-magnesium-should-i-take

Vitamin K2 Optimal Doses

As for magnesium, most people need to increase the amount of vitamin k2 they typically consume. Table II.5.1 below is given as a reference so that you can estimate the amount of vitamin K2 daily intake.

- for **50 kg** body weight and **4,500 IU** daily vitamin D3 supplementation; the vitamin K2 supplementation is **200 mcg** daily
- for **55 kg** body weight and **4,950 IU** daily vitamin D3 supplementation; the vitamin K2 supplementation is **220 mcg** daily
- for **60 kg** body weight and **5,400 IU** daily vitamin D3 supplementation; the vitamin K2 supplementation is **240 mcg** daily
- for **65 kg** body weight and **5,850 IU** daily vitamin D3 supplementation; the vitamin K2 supplementation is **260 mcg** daily
- for **70 kg** body weight and **6,300 IU** daily vitamin D3 supplementation; the vitamin K2 supplementation is **280 mcg** daily
- for **75 kg** body weight and **6,750 IU** daily vitamin D3 supplementation; the vitamin K2 supplementation is **300 mcg** daily
- for **80 kg** body weight and **7,200 IU** daily vitamin D3 supplementation; the vitamin K2 supplementation is **320 mcg** daily
- for **85 kg** body weight and **7,650 IU** daily vitamin D3 supplementation; the vitamin K2 supplementation is **340 mcg** daily
- for **90 kg** body weight and **8,100 IU** daily vitamin D3 supplementation; the vitamin K2 supplementation is **360 mcg** daily
- for **95 kg** body weight and **8,550 IU** daily vitamin D3 supplementation; the vitamin K2 supplementation is **380 mcg** daily
- for **100 kg** body weight and **9,000 IU** daily vitamin D3 supplementation; the vitamin K2 supplementation is **400**

mcg daily

- for **105 kg** body weight and **9,450 IU** daily vitamin D3 supplementation; the vitamin K2 supplementation is **420 mcg** daily
- for **110 kg** body weight and **9,900 IU** daily vitamin D3 supplementation; the vitamin K2 supplementation is **440 mcg** daily

table 2.5.1

For values that are not in the table, you have to use the extrapolation formula:

The estimated vitamin K2 dose (mcg) = multiply the calculated maintenance dose by 4.5 and divide by 100

Example 1:

- Subject: female, non-pregnant and non-lactating
- weight: 77 kg,
- The subject has a correct absorptive capacity,
- The subject has a BMI = 24.5 (normal)
- The calculated maintenance dose is: 6930 (roughly 7,000) IU daily intake
- The estimated vitamin K2 dose is extrapolated to **310 mcg.** Because for 75 kg body weight and 6,750 IU daily vitamin D3 supplementation, the vitamin K2 supplementation is 300 mcg daily, and for 80 kg body weight and 7,200 IU daily vitamin D3 supplementation, the vitamin K2 supplementation is 320 mcg daily

Example 2:

- Subject: female, non-pregnant and non-lactating
- weight: 59 kg,
- The subject has a correct absorptive capacity,

- The subject has a BMI = 20.5 (normal)
- The calculated maintenance dose is: 5310 (roughly 5,300) IU daily intake
- The estimated vitamin K2 dose is extrapolated to **240 mcg.** Because of 60 kg body weight and 5,400 IU daily vitamin D3 supplementation.

Example 3:

- Subject: female
- weight: 78 kg,
- The subject has a correct absorptive capacity,
- The subject has a BMI = 31 (obese)
- The calculated maintenance dose is: 7,020 IU daily intake
- The adjusted maintenance dose is: 8,424 (roughly 8,400) IU daily intake
- The estimated vitamin K2 dose is extrapolated based on the calculated maintenance dose (7,020 IU) and not the adjusted maintenance dose. The estimated vitamin K2 dose is extrapolated to **316 mcg.**

Additional factors to take into account

If you are taking medications that reduce the absorption of vitamin D, consider increasing your vitamin D intake by up to 20 percent. (see chapter "Factors Influencing Vitamin D Status")

If you are obese (body mass index (BMI) of 30) or have fat malabsorption syndrome, consider increasing your vitamin D intake by up to 20 percent.

To obtain the optimal vitamin D's beneficial effect on your bone health, you have to ingest, either from supplements or the diet, 1,000 milligrams of calcium a day if you are under fifty years and 1,200 milligrams of calcium if you are over fifty years.

Caution should be observed in patients with impairment of renal function, cardiovascular diseases, tuberculosis, or chronic fungal infections.

IV. If you have a serum vitamin D level higher than 110 nanograms/mL (p4)

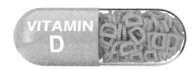

In this case, consider reducing your vitamin D intake to reach a vitamin D level in the range of 50-80 nanograms/mL (70-225 nmol/L). Levels equal to or higher than 150 nanograms/mL (375 nmol/mL) raise the problem of vitamin D toxicity which may occur when levels are over 200 nanograms/mL (500 nmol/mL).

14

FACTORS INFLUENCING VITAMIN D STATUS

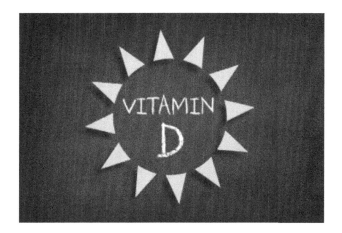

Various factors influence the photosynthesis efficiency and the bioavailability of vitamin D and contribute to the risk of inadequate vitamin D status (deficiency and insufficiency).

These factors include residence latitude, season, time of day, clothing, age, obesity, sunscreen use, skin type, and the incidence of some chronic illnesses.

Factors Influencing the Bioavailability of Vitamin D After Oral Ingestion or Cutaneous Production

The bioavailability of vitamin D is defined as the proportion of the ingested amount of vitamin D (total vitamin D in food), which ends up in systemic circulation. Thus, It is important to determine the major factors limiting the bioavailability of vitamin D acquired after oral ingestion or cutaneous synthesis.

Factors impacting the gastrointestinal absorption of vitamin D

Vitamin D seems to be absorbed in the gut from 55 to 99% depending on several factors. Its absorption occurs in the proximal small intestine and is influenced by stomach secretions, pancreatic secretions, biliary secretions, the integrity of the intestine wall, and the intestine's ability to absorb dietary fat.

- People with any condition that causes intestinal fat malabsorption may experience impaired vitamin D absorption. This susceptibility includes persons with untreated celiac disease, pancreatic enzyme insufficiency, bowel disease, and those who have had certain sections of their bowel removed.
- Individuals with the following conditions may have impaired vitamin D absorption: liver failure, pancreatic insufficiency, gastric bypass, Crohn's disease, untreated celiac disease, and cystic fibrosis
- Individuals taking bile acid sequestrants for hypercholesterolemia, such as colestyramine (Questran, Prevalite), colesevelam (Welchol), and colestipol (Colestid, Flavored Colestid), may experience impaired vitamin D absorption.

Obesity. Obesity is a severe health condition that may also be associated with poor cutaneous vitamin D production. Several studies evaluated the production of vitamin D3 following whole-body irradiation in obese and nonobese subjects. The circulating vitamin D [25(OH)D] levels in participants' blood showed that the resulting increase in vitamin D3 was 57 percent lower in obese than in nonobese subjects. Similar observations occurred after an oral dose of 50,000 IU of vitamin D.

The reason for this obesity-associated vitamin D deficiency is not clear, although the studies conducted. Some studies have suggested that the excess fat in obese patients absorbs and keeps the vitamin D trapped so that it cannot be used to mineralize the skeleton or maintain cellular health properly.

Bioavailability of Vitamin D2 and D3. Vitamin D2 and D3, as described in the chapter "The miraculous making of vitamin D," differ only in their side-chain structure. Physiological actions of these two steroid hormones include calcium and phosphorus homeostasis, cell cycling and proliferation4, cell differentiation5, and apoptosis6.

Early studies suggested these two forms of vitamin D as equipotent and interchangeable in humans. However, recent studies showed that **vitamin D2 was by far less effective than vitamin D3 in increasing the serum level of vitamin D [25(OH)D]**—the indicator of vitamin D insufficiency and deficiency in the blood—. One study in 2011 found that vitamin D3 (cholecalciferol) is 87 percent more potent than Vitamin D2 (ergocalciferol). Another study determined that the same single dose of vitamin D2 does not last longer than the dose of D3. In other terms, in humans, vitamin D3 provides greater benefits than vitamin D2. Therefore, vitamin D3 should be considered the preferred treatment or supplementation option.

Drugs that interfere with the absorption

Several drugs interfere with vitamin D metabolism by activating the pregnane X receptor, thereby causing vitamin D malabsorption and deficiency. Drugs that interfere with absorption are the following:

- antacids
- anti-inflammatory drugs - corticosteroids
- anti-cancer drugs (Taxol ® and related compounds)
- anticholesterol drugs (Cholestyramine ® and Colestipol ®)
- anticonvulsants (phenobarbital ®, carbamazepine ®, phenytoin ®)
- antifungals (Clotrimazole ®, Ketoconazole ®)
- antiretrovirals (AIDS therapies)
- bactericidal antibiotic (Rifampin ®)
- barbiturates (Phenobarbital ®)
- medicinal plants - St. John's Wort and its extracts (hypericin, hyperforin)

Factors influencing cutaneous vitamin D3 synthesis

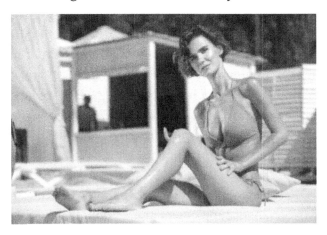

The production of vitamin D3 in human skin depends on the amount of ultraviolet B radiation reaching the dermis and the availability of 7-dehydrocholesterol. Thus, the amount of endogenously produced vitamin D is influenced by the following:

- factors that affect the number of ultraviolet B photons that

strike human skin like atmospheric components, geographic location, season, time of day, clothing, sunscreen use, and skin pigmentation
- factors that influence the availability of 7-dehydrocholesterol, including age, obesity, and the impact of some chronic illnesses.

Geographic location. In the northern hemisphere, during the summer season, the radiations from the sun hit the earth's surface more directly than at any other season. Ultraviolet B radiation that hits the skin is maximal, and you can get the most sun and UVB penetration.

When the zenith angle is more oblique, the Ultraviolet B radiation traverses a long path through the stratospheric ozone layer, which decreases the number of UVB radiation reaching the earth's surface. That is the explanation the skin produces little if any, vitamin D3 from the sun at latitudes above 37° north or below 37° (degrees) south of the equator when the solar rays are more oblique during the autumn and winter months.

During winter, Northern Hemisphere is tilted away from the sun, and the angle that sunlight passes through the atmosphere is more oblique.

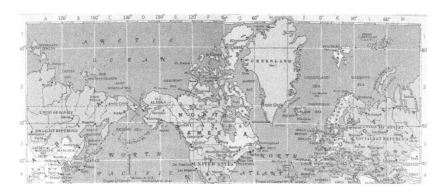

People who live above the 37-degree latitude line —roughly the imaginary line between Philadelphia and San Francisco— (in the United States, the shaded region in the map) are at greater risk for vitamin D deficiency during the autumn and winter months. Under these circumstances, to achieve vitamin D adequacy without sun exposure, people must take vitamin D3 supplements and/or fortified food.

Type of Skin. Human skin color displays variations throughout life and is influenced by several factors such as race, age, sex, and hormones. However, the most important factors that determine human skin color are the quantity of melanin pigment and its chemical structure. Melanin, the pigment responsible for the difference in skin color among racial groups, acts as a powerful natural sunscreen that efficiently absorbs solar-UVB photons and thus substantially diminishes the production of vitamin D3 in the skin.

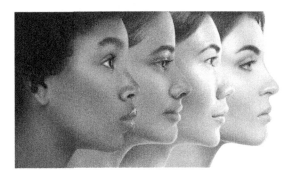

This inhibitory effect on Cutaneous Vitamin D production increases with skin color. Hence, dark-skinned people require more sunlight exposure than fair or light-skinned people to produce an equivalent vitamin D.

Sunscreens use. Sunscreens prevent sunburn, skin aging, and skin cancer by blocking UVB light. A sunscreen with a sun protection factor of 15 (SPF 15) filters 93 percent of UVB rays and thus reduces vitamin D3 biosynthesis by the same degree.

SPF 30 Sunscreens filter 97 percent of UVB photons, and SPF 50 blocks out 98 percent. That leaves only from 2 to 7 percent of solar-

UVB reaching human skin, consequently decreasing vitamin D3 biosynthesis.

Age. Researchers conducted an extensive evaluation of surgically obtained skin (age range between 8 and 92 years) to identify if the cutaneous production of vitamin D3 is age-dependent. Skins were exposed to ultraviolet radiation, and the contents of previtamin D3 were determined in the epidermis and dermis.

The researchers found that aging can significantly decrease the capacity of the skin to produce previtamin D3 (by $\geq$ twofold).

Compared with younger, the elderly have lower levels of the 7-dehydrocholesterol in the skin that ultraviolet B light converts into the previtamin D3.

PART III

PART III

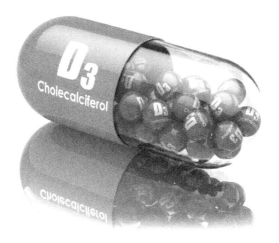

15

PREGNANCY, LACTATION AND VITAMIN D

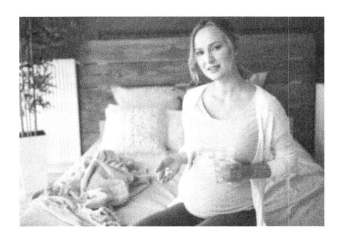

Vitamin D deficiency is very common among pregnant women and increases the risk of gestational diabetes mellitus, preeclampsia, and preterm birth. Severe maternal vitamin D deficiency is linked with disordered bone homeostasis, congenital rickets, and fractures in the newborn. Expecting mothers need to get sufficient amounts of Vitamin D to raise their vitamin D [25(OH)D] to the range of 40—60 nanograms/mL (100—150 nmol/L), thus improving maternal and infant health outcomes.

Emerging scientific and clinical literature currently exists for vitamin D and pregnancy due to the increasing awareness of the association between vitamin D adequacy and maternal and infant health outcomes. PUBMED (The National Library of Medicine) lists ≥ 5,154 publications that use the keywords "**vitamin D**" and "**pregnancy**" in either the title or abstract from 1932 to the present, with most of the research published in the last decade. This total includes publications that combine the use of the terms "vitamin D" and "pregnancy" with one of the following terms:

- women (≥ 2,392 publications)
- infant (≥ 1,682 publications),
- newborn (≥ 1,177 publications),
- child (≥ 1,582 publications),
- women (≥ 2,392 publications),
- lactation (≥ 763 publications),
- preeclampsia (≥ 438 publications)
- loss (≥ 236 publications)

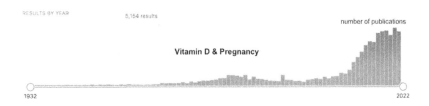

figure 3.1.1: increase in the number of articles published each year with the terms "pregnancy" and "vitamin D" in the title or abstract (in PUBMED.)

Knowledge of vitamin D in the health of pregnant women, infants, and children has grown substantially over the years, extending the importance of vitamin D to non-classical functions. Vitamin D has non-classical effects that may influence other aspects of pregnant women, lactating women, infants, and young child health. Growing and emerging studies have pointed out the role of optimal vitamin D status on positive pregnancy and infant health outcomes. Vitamin D regulates the innate immune system1 to produce more effective antiviral, antibacterial, and anti-inflammatory effects. It also modulates the responses of the adaptive immune system to prevent autoimmunity diseases such as type 1 diabetes. Vitamin D also produces, through several mechanisms, positive outcomes on brain development and behavior well before the child's birth.

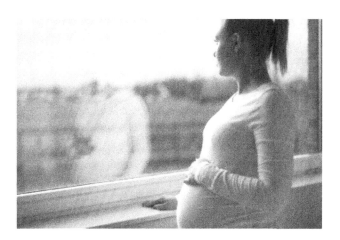

Recent studies show that many beneficial vitamin D effects on young child health begin in the first months of pregnancy and are associated with optimal maternal vitamin D status. Conversely, severe maternal vitamin D deficiency has been linked to poor newborn health outcomes, including skeletal disorders, congenital rickets, motor development delay, and muscle weakness.

So, even if routine screening for vitamin D deficiency is not recommended for pregnant women, and considering the effects of adequate supplementation in producing positive maternal and fetal outcomes. It is strongly recommended that each pregnant woman be assessed for vitamin D deficiency and supplemented for the most satisfactory health outcome for the newborn and the pregnant mother.

Preeclampsia (gestational hypertension)

Preeclampsia is a pregnancy complication with severe consequences that can happen about midway through pregnancy. Mild for most pregnant women, it can become severe for others.

Women with preeclampsia experience high blood pressure and are at increased risk of developing diseases affecting the brain, kidneys, liver, and brain. Preeclampsia may also affect the placenta and cause severe health problems for the infant.

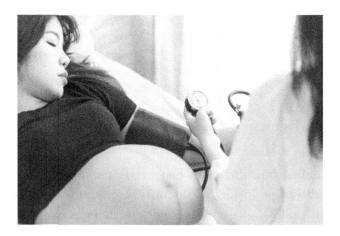

Several meta-analyses of observational studies have established a strong association between low vitamin D status and adverse pregnancy outcomes such as gestational diabetes, preeclampsia, birth weight, and preterm birth.

Most recently, clinical studies have shown that the prescription of vitamin D supplements in the first trimester of pregnancy prevents the development of preeclampsia.

Gestational diabetes

Gestational diabetes develops during pregnancy in women who don't already have diabetes. Managing gestational diabetes will help ensure a healthy pregnancy and a healthy baby. Gestational diabetes, present in 7–14% of pregnancies in the United States, increases your risk of developing preeclampsia or high blood pressure that causes unsatisfactory maternal and infant health outcomes.

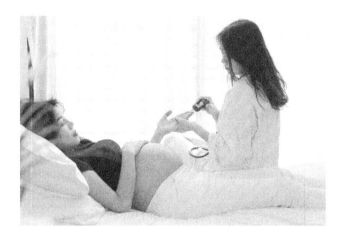

Several observational studies have found that low vitamin D [25(OH)D] level is linked with an increased risk of gestational diabetes mellitus.

During pregnancy, vitamin D supplementation improves maternal vitamin D status and enhances insulin sensitivity and glucose tolerance.

The American College of Obstetrics and Gynecology has suggested that monitoring may be considered for pregnant women at high risk for vitamin D deficiency, and if pregnant women are found to be deficient, then supplementation with 1000–2000 IU is recommended.

However, newer data suggests supplementing 4000 to 5000 IU vitamin D for pregnant women, administered daily during six months of pregnancy. (10,000 IU per day is the most conservative safety threshold)

Vitamin D Status during Pregnancy

The pregnant woman experiences significant physical, physiological, and emotional changes to nurture and accommodate the developing fetus. During pregnancy, she is responsible for her health and her developing fetus and thus has to consider lifestyle and diet that promotes positive pregnancy outcomes.

As vitamin D plays an important role in general fetal growth and development, including fetal skeletal development and tooth enamel formation, the pregnant mother should achieve an optimal vitamin D status. Conversely, If a pregnant woman has a low vitamin D status, she is at increased risk of severe pregnancy complications. As her fetus depends on the maternal supply of vitamin D, a deficiency is associated with smaller birth sizes and an increased risk of common childhood diseases, such as asthma and type 1 diabetes.

With all the available evidence regarding vitamin D supplementation for pregnant women, and taking into account the benefits of supplementation in producing positive maternal and fetal outcomes and the adverse and harmful effects of low vitamin D status in both pregnant women and infants, we consider that achieving a **circulating level of 25(OH)D in the range of 40—60 nanograms/mL (100—150 nmol/L) during pregnancy** is considered as adequate for improving fetal development and preventing maternal complications.

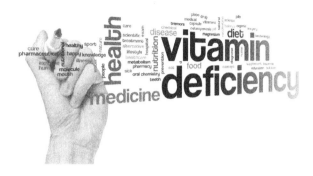

Vitamin D deficiency in pregnant women should be corrected in the same way as in nonpregnant women. Daily doses of 4000 units/day have already been recommended for vitamin D correction in pregnancy and are considered safe. (for more details, please refer to chapter 5: "Vitamin D Optimal Doses," Part II)

A growing body of evidence has established that vitamin D3 supplementation during pregnancy improves maternal and infant circulating vitamin D [25(OH)D] levels. Thus, supplementation benefits the pregnant mother and infant, improves maternal insulin sensitivity, and promotes fetal growth. Evidence was strong that vitamin D supplementation produces positive health outcomes for pregnant women by significantly decreasing maternal insulin resistance and reducing the risk of preeclampsia (gestational diabetes). The health outcomes of maternal vitamin D supplementation for the infant include normal measures of fetal size, normal body composition, and good skeletal mineralization, in addition to a lower risk of developing diabetes type 1 and asthma.

Vitamin D Deficiency and early childhood

Your child's bones and teeth need sufficient calcium and phosphorous to develop properly. And it is vitamin D that ensures that the bones and teeth get enough calcium and phosphorus. Without enough vitamin D, bones remain soft and weak and may bend or have an abnormal shape. Calcium is also important for the normal functioning of every cell in your child's body. This helps us understand why Vitamin D is important for your baby's healthy growth and well-being and how its deficiency will affect them.

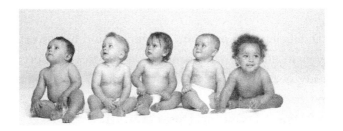

The benefits of achieving optimal status during pregnancy and lactation may protect the mother against adverse pregnancy outcomes and improve maternal and neonatal outcomes.

- lower risk of gestational diabetes
- lower risk of preeclampsia
- reduced risk of preterm birth
- reduced risk of neonatal deaths
- lower risk of low birth weight
- reduced risk of rickets in babies
- reduced risk of muscle weakness
- reduced risk of motor developmental delay

However, combined vitamin D and calcium supplementing represents an increased risk of preterm birth. The supervision of the clinician is highly recommended.

Lactation and optimal vitamin D status

When breastfeeding, you produce milk with a certain amount of vitamin D, depending on your vitamin D status.

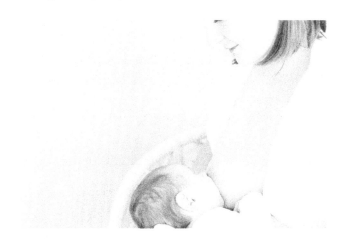

Recent studies have shown that lactating women with a vitamin D [25(OH)D] levels equal to or higher than 20 nanograms/mL (50 nmol/L) and taking a daily vitamin D supplementation in the range of 400 to 2,000 IU produces milk concentrations insufficient to deliver the daily vitamin D needed to an exclusively breastfed infant. Maternal milk is also considered inadequate to correct pre-existing infant low vitamin D status through breastfeeding alone.

The same studies have established that breastfeeding mothers must get a minimum vitamin D dosage equal to or higher than 4,000 IU to produce milk with vitamin D levels sufficient for the daily infant need. However, this adequate intake of vitamin D during pregnancy and lactation of 4,000 IU/ day is grossly inadequate because, based on the hypothesis that the cutoff point of vitamin D sufficiency during pregnancy is 20 nanograms/mL (50 nmol/L).

As we consider that the optimal vitamin D status corresponds to serum vitamin D [25(OH)D] concentrations in the range of 40—60 nanograms/mL (100—150 nmol/L), lactating women may consider reaching the optimal D status in this range by increasing their vitamin D daily intakes accordingly. (please refer to the chapter "Vitamin D Optimal Doses," Part II, for more detailed information)

A circulating level of 25(OH)D in the range of 40—60 nanograms/mL (100—150 nmol/L) during pregnancy and lactation is considered adequate for improving fetal development and preventing maternal complications. (please refer to the chapter "Vitamin D Optimal Doses," Part II, for more detailed information)

Babies may need a vitamin D boost

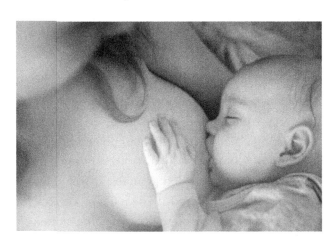

Breastfed babies and babies born prematurely need vitamin D supplementation because a typical mother's breast milk does not give her baby enough vitamin D. There are two ways to achieve that:

- The baby can be directly given 400 to 1000 IU drops a day.
- Or the mother can take 5,000 to 10,000 IU a day (1,0000 IU is the most conservative safety threshold), fortifying breast milk with sufficient vitamin D for the baby.

Although all standard infant formulas are fortified, vitamin D supplementation is recommended for formula-fed babies due to insufficient vitamin D in infant formula.

Vitamin D Supplementation — The Optimal Doses

Your starting point is to check your vitamin D [25(OH)D] level in the blood and refer to the next paragraph to identify your vitamin D status.

Expecting mothers need to get sufficient amounts of Vitamin D to raise their serum vitamin D [25(OH)D] to the range of 40—60 nanograms/mL (100—150 nmol/L), thus improving maternal and infant health outcomes.

Please refer to the chapter "vitamin D optimal doses" in Part II for detailed information on achieving your desired vitamin D status.

16

CANCER AND VITAMIN D

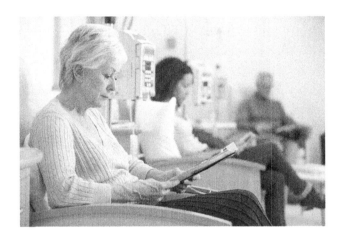

Vitamin D exerts antiproliferative actions and promotes cellular death on malignant cells. A convergent body of evidence has emerged from epidemiology and clinical trials that associate adequate vitamin D levels (50—80 nanograms/mL) with decreased risk of developing certain cancers and better cancer treatment outcomes by increasing apoptosis in malignant cells. Recent studies linked a 4 nanograms/mL (10 nmol/L) increase in circulating vitamin D [25(OH)D] levels to a 4 percent increase in survival among cancer patients.

Cancer is a major cause of death in the world, accounting for nearly 10 million deaths in 2020. Cancer is marked by the rapid creation of malignant cells that grow beyond their usual boundaries and which can, with time, spread to other organs.

The predominant methods of cancer treatment are surgery, chemotherapy, and irradiation. Depending on the type and stage of cancer, these methods can be provided in combination. Though early treatment can lead to total remission in many cancers, early diagnosis is not possible in most cases.

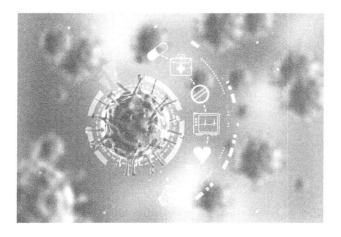

An enormous body of scientific and clinical literature on vitamin D and cancers currently exists. PUBMED (National Library of Medicine) lists ≥ 12,690 publications using the keywords "vitamin D" and "cancer" in either the title or abstract from 1946 to the present. This total includes articles that combine the use of *vitamin D* with one of the following terms:

- *cancer* treatment (≥ 7,318 articles),
- *cancer* prevention (≥ 3,534 articles),

- *breast cancer* (≥ 2,066 articles),
- *prostate cancer* (≥1,465),
- *colon* cancer (≥842),
- *lung* cancer (≥488),
- *ovarian cancer* (≥298).

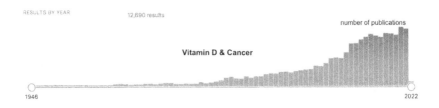

figure 3.1.1: increase in the number of articles published each year with the term cancer and vitamin D in the title or abstract (in PUBMED.)

Finally, PUBMED lists ≥4,583 publications with the term *calcitriol and cancer* in the title or abstract, ≥5701 articles with *vitamin D3* and cancer, and ≥402 articles with *vitamin D2 and cancer*.

———

The newer scientific studies and clinical knowledge support that an optimal supplementation of vitamin D may lead to better outcomes in preventing cancer, reducing its incidence, and improving survival rates. In a 2009 study, the authors established that raising the minimum year-around vitamin D [25(OH)D] level to 40—60 ng/mL (100—150 nmol/L) would prevent each year nearly 58,000 cases of breast cancer and 50,000 cases of colorectal cancer, and three-fourths of deaths from these cancers in the United States and Canada.

The discovery that many tissues and cells in the human body, including, among others, the brain, skin, colon, breast, and prostate, have an enzymatic process that is similar to the kidneys in converting

25(OH)D to 1,25(OH)2D, provided new knowledge on how vitamin D could have other health benefits and improve cancer, cardiovascular diseases, and autoimmune disorders outcomes significantly.

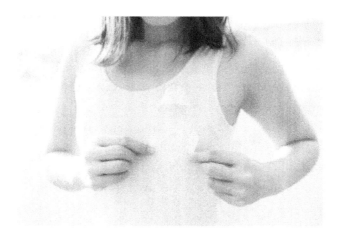

Local production of active vitamin D [1,25(OH)2D] in the breast, colon, prostate and other cells regulates various genes that control proliferation and apoptosis —the process of programmed cell death to eliminate unwanted cells.

Many studies have shown that vitamin D adequacy is associated with beneficial effects on reducing the incidence, severity, and risk of breast, prostate, colon, and ovarian cancer. Several studies identified a protective relationship between adequate vitamin D levels in the blood and reduced cancer risk. Thus, optimal vitamin D supplementation may substantially reduce the risk of developing certain types of cancer and lower their incidence with no adverse effects.

In malignancies, vitamin D levels that produce good outcomes are expected to be high. Epidemiological evidence regarding **vitamin D [25(OH)D] has shown that levels in the range of 50-80 nanograms/mL are associated with a reduced risk of developing many common cancers such as breast, colon, prostate, and ovarian cancer.**

Recent observational studies have also demonstrated that colorectal cancer risk is at its lowest point for a vitamin D [25(OH)D] level equal to 55 nanograms/mL (137 nmol/L). Vitamin D [25(OH)D] range of 50 and 80 nanograms/mL (125 and 200 nmol/L)

The Anti-cancer Actions of Vitamin D

Through Vitamin D Receptors located in practically every human body cell, hormonally active vitamin D regulates the activities of more than 200 genes mainly involved in cell cycling and proliferation, differentiation, and apoptosis. In other words, the active form of vitamin D has physiological functions, including regulating the growth and differentiation of a large part of normal and malignant cells. Active vitamin D plays a protective role against cancer by:

1. decreasing the multiplication of malignant cells
2. reducing the risk of proliferation of these cells by reducing the vascularization of cancer cells.
3. inhibiting the transformation of precancerous cells into cancerous cells
4. inducing the death of cancer cells (apoptosis) to some extent. If a cell begins to behave abnormally and is in the phase of becoming a malignant cell, activated vitamin D influences specific genes to inhibit cell growth or induce apoptosis (cell death).

Breast cancer

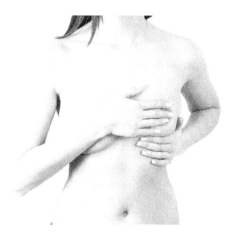

Breast cancer is the 2nd most common cancer diagnosed in women in the United States after skin cancer. Breast cancer evolves silently; however, mammograms can detect it early before spreading.

Breast cancer is a disease in which abnormal cells in the breast grow and divide out of control. Although breast cancer can start in different parts of the breast, it begins mainly in the lobules or the ducts. There are different kinds of breast cancers depending on which cells in the breast turn into cancer. When cancer spreads to other parts of the patient's body, it is said to have metastasized.

Symptoms

While the majority of patients experience different symptoms of breast cancer, others do not have any symptoms at all.

Symptoms of breast cancer include:

- New lump in the breast or armpits.
- Irritation or dimpling of the skin of the breast
- Nipple discharges other than breast milk, including blood.
- irritation or dimpling of breast skin.
- Pain in any area of the breast.
- Changes in the size and/or shape of the breast.

The type of treatment a patient has for breast cancer depends on the stage of their cancer. Treatments include surgery, chemotherapy, radiotherapy, and hormonal therapy.

Vitamin D's role in breast cancer

Several studies have shown the association between vitamin D status and breast cancer risk. Women with the highest levels of circulating vitamin D [25(OH)D] were less likely to develop breast cancer compared with women with the lowest level of circulating vitamin D [25(OH)D] (about a 45% decrease in breast cancer risk). Other studies have demonstrated that women with circulating vitamin D [25(OH)D] levels below 30 nanograms/mL (75 nmol/L) are at a higher risk of breast cancer.

A 2018 observational study has established that women aged 55 years of age or older with a vitamin D [25(OH)D] level equal to or greater than 60 nanograms/mL (150 nmol/L) had an 80 percent reduced risk of breast cancer when compared to women with a vitamin D [25(OH)D] level equal or lower than 20 nanograms/mL (50 nmol/L).

In addition, some observational studies have shown that women who were vitamin D-deficient at the time of their breast cancer diagnosis had worse outcomes, including higher rates of recurrence and increased risk of death from their cancers.

An optimal blood level of circulating vitamin D [25(OH)D] in the range of 50—80 nanograms/mL (125—200 nmol/L) may prevent breast cancer, improve the efficacy of chemotherapy and improve long-term survival for breast cancer patients.

Ovarian cancer

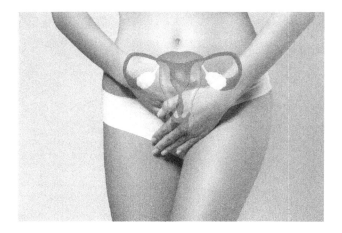

Ovarian cancer, also known as cancer of the ovaries, is a type of cancer that begins in the ovaries. The ovaries are pair of small organs located in the female reproductive system. The ovaries produce eggs as well as the hormones—estrogen and progesterone. Ovarian cancer begins when abnormal cells in the ovary grow and divide out of control.

Although ovarian cancer may develop at any age, it is more common in women who have been through menopause (older than 50 years).

Symptoms

Cancer of the ovaries may cause several symptoms, including:

- Bloating
- Back pain
- Pelvic or abdominal pain
- Lack of appetite or feeling full quickly
- Pain during sex
- Constipation
- Irregular menstrual cycles

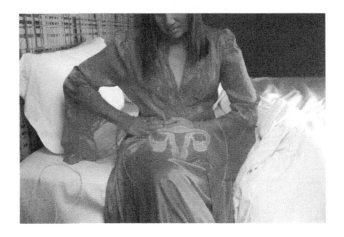

The treatment of ovarian cancer generally involves a combination of surgery and chemotherapy.

Although the five-year survival rate for the cancer of the ovaries has improved significantly in the past two decades, the prognosis remains poor overall, with a roughly 48% 5-year relative survival rate.

Vitamin D's role in ovarian cancer

Epidemiological evidence suggests that low vitamin **D status is linked to higher ovarian cancer risk.** Furthermore, recent observational studies have found that higher circulating vitamin D [25(OH)D] levels at diagnosis have been found to promote more prolonged survival among women with the disease.

An optimal blood level of circulating vitamin D [25(OH)D] in the range of 50—80 nanograms/mL (125—200 nmol/L) may increase the survival chance among women with ovarian cancer substantially.

Colorectal (colon) cancer

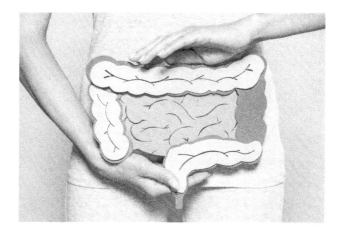

Colorectal cancer (colon cancer, rectum cancer) is the 3rd most common cancer in the United States and the second cause of cancer-related deaths.

Colorectal (colon) cancer is a disease in which abnormal colon or rectum cells grow out of control.

Most colorectal cancers start as polyps, which are small abnormal tissue growths in the colon lining. Most polyps are nonmalignant; however, some polyps, known as adenomatous or adenomas, may grow uncontrollably and become cancerous over time.

Colorectal polyps and colorectal cancer are silent and always don't cause symptoms early. Periodical screening tests are crucial because they can find polyps early to be removed before turning into cancer. Even when polyps become malignant, screening allows early diagnosis and treatment.

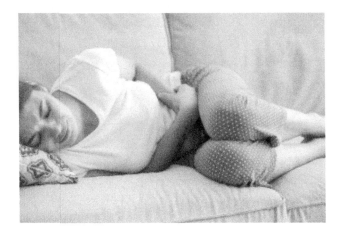

Symptoms

Colorectal cancer may cause several symptoms, including:

- Symptoms of colorectal cancer may include:
- Continued change in bowel habits (diarrhea or constipation, feeling of incomplete stool evacuation)
- Blood in or on the stool (black or bright red stools)
- Abdominal pain or cramps that don't go away
- Bloating
- Bleeding after a bowel movement;
- Unexplained weight loss;
- Grand fatigue.

The primary and first treatment for colorectal cancer is surgery to remove the malignant tumors, followed by chemotherapy. Radiation therapy may also be indicated to treat rectal cancer.

Vitamin D's role in colorectal cancer

Recent studies have established a stronger association between circulating vitamin D [25(OH)D] levels and the incidence of polyps and adenomas in the colon. High levels of circulating vitamin D [25(OH)D] are linked with a reduced risk of developing polyps or adenomas in the colon and rectum due to the regulatory effect of vitamin D in cell proliferation and differentiation, cell growth, and cell death. The active vitamin D alters the expression of the genes that regulate the growth, differentiation, and survival of polyps cells in the colon.

Optimal vitamin D status produces better colorectal cancer outcomes, including the overall survival of colon cancer patients.

Observational studies have demonstrated that **colorectal cancer risk is at its lowest point for a vitamin D [25(OH)D] level equal to 55 nanograms/mL (137 nmol/L).** Vitamin D [25(OH)D] level in the range of 50 and 80 nanograms/mL (125 and 200 nmol/L) is considered optimal in reducing the risk of developing colorectal cancer.

Vitamin D Supplementation — The Optimal Doses

Your starting point is to check your vitamin D [25(OH)D] level in the blood and refer to the next paragraph to identify your vitamin D status.

The optimal vitamin D [25(OH)D] level is between 50 and 80 nanograms/mL (125 to 200 nmol/L), which corresponds to the preventive cancer range based on strong evidence about the association between vitamin D and beneficial health outcomes, including cancer prevention, and treatment of some conditions including Psoriatic arthritis, asthma, rheumatoid arthritis, and tuberculosis.

Please refer to the chapter "vitamin D optimal doses" in Part II for detailed information on achieving your desired vitamin D status.

17

CARDIOVASCULAR DISEASES AND VITAMIN D

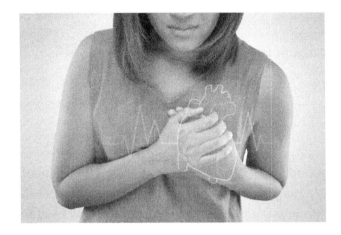

Heart and blood vessel disease include multiple conditions, many of which are linked to atherosclerosis.

Atherosclerosis is a disease that develops when plaques build up in the inner lining of an artery. Plaques are made up of a combination of fatty substances deposits, cholesterol, waste products from cells, calcium, and a clotting agent (fibrin).

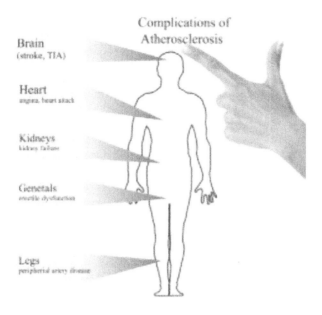

This buildup of plaque with time narrows the arteries, making it hard for blood to flow through. This buildup can occur in any artery around your heart, brain, and kidneys. If a blood clot forms, it can dangerously block the blood flow and cause a stroke or heart attack.

Cardiovascular diseases (CVD) or heart diseases are heart and blood vessel disorders. They include:

Heart attack

A heart attack—also called a myocardial infarction—occurs when a clot stops the blood flow to a part of the heart. The blockage is most often caused by plaques in the arteries that feed the heart and might be complete or partial. A complete blockage of an artery implies the patient developed an ST-elevation myocardial infarction ("STEMI" heart attack). In this case, the part supplied by that artery of the heart muscle begins to die and requires immediate care to restore the blood flow quickly to the damaged part of the heart muscle. "STEMI" heart attack is the most severe and dangerous form of heart attack and requires emergency assessment and treatment. In contrast, a partial blockage is called a non-ST-elevation myocardial infarction ("NSTEMI" heart attack). Any heart attack is a life-threatening medical condition that requires emergency assessment and treatment.

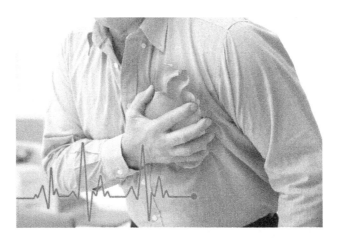

Heart attack

A heart attack—also called a myocardial infarction—occurs when a clot stops the blood flow to a part of the heart. The blockage is most often caused by plaques in the arteries that feed the heart and might be complete or partial. A complete blockage of an artery implies the patient developed an ST-elevation myocardial infarction ("STEMI" heart attack). In this case, the part supplied by that artery of the heart muscle begins to die and requires immediate care to restore the blood flow quickly to the damaged part of the heart muscle. "STEMI" heart attack is the most severe and dangerous form of heart attack and requires emergency assessment and treatment. In contrast, a partial blockage is called a non-ST-elevation myocardial infarction ("NSTEMI" heart attack). Any heart attack is a life-threatening medical condition that requires emergency assessment and treatment.

Common heart attack symptoms include:

- chest pain or discomfort.
- discomfort and/or pain in one or both arms or shoulders.
- discomfort and/or pain in the jaw.
- discomfort and/or pain in the neck.
- discomfort and/or pain in the back.
- discomfort and/or pain in the stomach.
- feeling of dizziness
- shortness of breath or trouble breathing.
- feeling of nausea or sickness

Several risk factors raise the probability of having a heart attack. This include:

- age. the heart attack risk increases with age
- family history,
- genetic or congenital conditions. Some genetic medical disorders can increase the heart attack risk,
- unhealthy diet, including a high intake of sodium, sugar, or fat,
- smoking and drinking too much alcohol,
- poor level of physical activity,
- particular drug abuse (e.g., amphetamines, cocaine).

Stroke

Stroke—one of the most dangerous and severe medical conditions — is a leading cause of severe disability and death for adults in the United States, with around 800,000 people developing stroke each year. Stroke is a cerebrovascular illness that affects the blood vessels that supply the brain with oxygen. When the brain doesn't receive sufficient oxygen, damage starts to occur. A stroke is a life-threatening medical condition that requires emergency assessment and treatment.

There are three main types of stroke:

- ischemic stroke—the most common type— occurs when the blood supplying the brain is stopped or reduced.
- hemorrhagic stroke develops when a blood vessel in the brain ruptures due to high blood pressure.
- transient ischemic attack (TIA) happens when the blood flow—to a part of the brain—is inadequate for a short period.

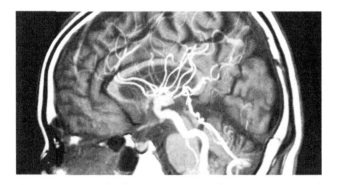

Common stroke symptoms include:

- weakness or numbness that occurs suddenly in the arm.
- weakness or numbness that occurs suddenly in the face.
- weakness or numbness that occurs suddenly in the leg.

- confusion, difficulty understanding speech or trouble speaking that occurs suddenly.
- trouble of vision that occurs suddenly.
- trouble walking, loss of balance, or lack of coordination that occurs suddenly.

Heart failure

Heart failure is a leading medical condition in the United States, affecting nearly 6 million Americans. Heart failure implies the heart cannot pump the body's blood correctly. The heart begins working but not as well as it should, causing the body's need for blood and oxygen not to be met.

The most common symptoms of this severe medical condition include:

- breathlessness during daily activities or at rest
- difficulties breathing when lying down
- fatigue
- swollen ankles and legs

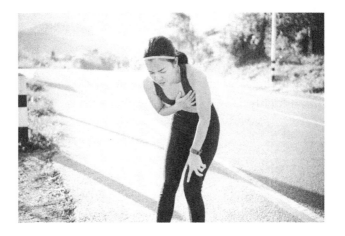

Other symptoms of heart failure may include:

- fast heart rate.
- persistent cough, getting worse at night,
- loss of appetite,
- weight gain or weight loss,
- dizziness and fainting,
- confusion,
- depression and anxiety

Heart failure treatment

Early diagnosis and treatment may reduce the incidence of heart failure and lower its severity. Treatment usually involves:

- Lifestyle changes.

- Taking a combination of medications.

- Surgical procedures.

- The use of specific devices.

High blood pressure

High blood pressure—also called hypertension, is a severe medical condition that raises the risks of heart disease, strokes, kidney damage, and other diseases.

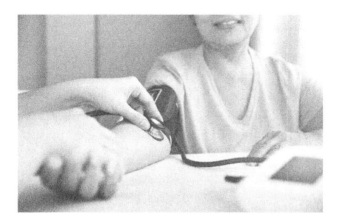

Blood pressure varies throughout the day based on your activities. It refers to the force exerted by the blood circulating against the walls of the body's arteries. Two numbers express blood pressure. The top number refers to the systolic or upper pressure and measures the tension in the arteries when your heart beats. The bottom number refers to the diastolic or lower pressure representing the vessels' pressure when your heart rests between beats.

Having blood pressure measures consistently > 130 mmHg for systolic and > 80 mmHg for diastolic results in the diagnosis of high blood pressure—hypertension.

The common risk factors include:

- unhealthy diets and eating habits—excessive salt consumption, high intake of saturated fat and trans fats, excessive coffee and tea consumption, low intake of fruits and vegetables

- bad lifestyle habits (poor physical activity, consumption of tobacco and alcohol)
- obesity
- family history of hypertension
- some medical conditions (e.g., diabetes or kidney disease)
- age over 65
- adverse effects of some medications

Symptoms of High blood pressure

Hypertension is usually silent and has no warning signs or symptoms —and most people do not know they have it. So, It is essential that you regularly measure your blood pressure to detect hypertension.

When symptoms begin, they may include

- headaches
- blurred vision
- nosebleeds
- irregular heart rhythms
- shortness of breath
- buzzing in the ears
- dizziness

Severe hypertension may cause:

- chest pain
- muscle tremors
- extreme fatigue,
- nausea and vomiting,
- confusion,
- anxiety.

Medications for high blood pressure

There are several medicines available for reducing blood pressure. Your doctor will offer you the appropriate medication. Drugs include:

- diuretics
- alpha-blockers and beta-blockers
- central agonists
- vasodilators
- calcium-channel blockers
- peripheral adrenergic inhibitor
- angiotensin receptor blockers
- angiotensin-converting enzyme inhibitors

Complications of untreated hypertension

Hypertension may cause severe damage to the heart, kidneys, brain, and other organs, including:

- heart attack
- strokes
- heart failure
- angina
- kidney failure

Cardiovascular Diseases and Vitamin D

Much scientific and clinical literature currently exists on vitamin D and pregnancy due to the increasing awareness of the association between vitamin D adequacy and maternal and infant health outcomes. PUBMED (The National Library of Medicine, and the first source for biomedical literature) lists ≥ 7,510 publications that use the keywords "**vitamin D**" and "**cardiovascular disease**" in either the title or abstract from 1947 to the present, with most of the researches published in the last decade. This total includes publications that combine the use of the terms "vitamin D" and "pregnancy" with one of the following terms:

- treatment (≥ 4,186 publications),
- deficiency (≥ 3,272 publications)
- prevention (≥ 2,332 publications)
- hypertension (≥ 1,642 publications),
- supplementation (≥ 1,503 publications),
- heart failure (≥ 739 publications),
- atherosclerosis (≥ 734 publications),
- heart failure (≥ 739 publications),
- stroke (≥ 543 publications)
- pregnancy (≥ 238 publications)

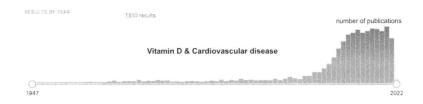

figure 3.1.1: increase in the number of articles published each year with the terms "cardiovascular disease" and "vitamin D" in the title or abstract (in PUBMED.)

Vitamin D has been identified as one of the most important factors in cardiovascular health due to its effects on various tissues and organs participating in atherosclerosis and its regulatory effects in this systemic inflammatory process. Through the Vitamin D Receptors (VDR) found practically in all organs and tissues involved in atherosclerosis development, vitamin D exerts at least two main effects critical for cardiovascular health.

Several epidemiological investigations have shown the protective effect of vitamin D against cardiovascular disease. In one study, a vitamin D [25(OH)D] level of fewer than 30 nanograms/mL (75 nmol/L) is linked with hypertension, diabetes, and hyperlipidemia in two-thirds of patients. This corresponds to an increased risk of developing heart disease compared with patients with vitamin D [25(OH)D] levels equal to and higher than 30 nanograms/mL (75 nmol/L).

Initial prospective studies have suggested a strong association between vitamin D [25(OH)D] levels and clinical cardiovascular disease events. Low vitamin D [25(OH)D] levels produce poor outcomes, particularly in individuals with preexisting CVD. Vitamin D deficiency —vitamin D [25(OH)D] lower than 30 nanograms/mL (75 nmol/L) was found to increase the risk of developing sudden cardiac death, heart failure, or incident hypertension significantly.

More recently, the role of vitamin D in attenuating inflammations has been scrutinized in cardiology due to the recent identification that inflammation is the most critical factor in promoting the formation and growth of plaque and arterial disease. Vitamin D is known for its essential role in preventing and treating inflammations through two separate mechanisms: regulating the formation of inflammatory cytokines and inhibiting the proliferation of pro-inflammatory cells. Thus, the identification that cardiac patients have higher levels of plasma homocysteine level (a biomarker of inflammation) than healthy people support the use of vitamin D supplementation to decrease the risk of strokes, heart attacks, hypertension, and maybe reverse heart disease.

Vitamin D Supplementation — The Optimal Doses

Assessment of vitamin D supplementation for many chronic diseases and disease prevention has been a subject of growing interest in recent years. Many studies have established the efficacy of vitamin D supplementation in preventing or treating many chronic diseases, such as cardiovascular disease, diabetes Mellitus, bone disorders, and cancer. The optimal doses and the step-by-step protocol to improve your vitamin D status are presented in the chapter "vitamin D optimal doses." This will allow you to get the full benefits of vitamin D and experience good health outcomes.

Maintaining an adequate vitamin D status between 40 and 60 nanograms/mL (100 to 150 nmol/L) for both women and men will significantly reduce the risk of incident hypertension, strokes, sudden cardiac death, and heart failure.

Your starting point is to check your vitamin D [25(OH)D] level in the blood and refer to the next paragraph to identify your vitamin D status.

Please refer to the chapter "vitamin D optimal doses" in Part II for detailed information on achieving your desired vitamin D status.

18

CHRONIC INFLAMMATORY DISEASES

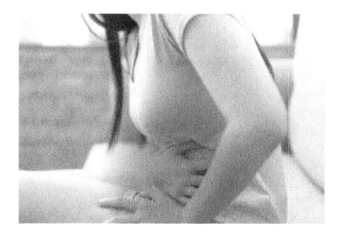

There is a growing interest in vitamin D as a potential treatment for several chronic inflammatory diseases. Besides its role in calcium homeostasis, vitamin D has essential effects in immunomodulation and modulating propensity to infection. Optimal vitamin D status in the 40-60 nanograms/mL range may improve chronic inflammation symptoms and outcomes.

Inflammation is a normal and protective response of the body against harmful stimuli such as bacteria, viruses, fungi, toxins, and physical trauma.

Inflammation is characterized by activating immune and non-immune cells to protect the body from harmful stimuli by eliminating infectious microorganisms and promoting recovery and tissue repair. Thus, the right kind of inflammation plays an essential role in healing, injury repair, and pathogens elimination to keep your body safe and healthy.

There are two kinds of inflammation acute and chronic. Acute inflammation is the body's immediate and immune response to harmful stimuli from infection, physical trauma, or stress. Acute inflammation is easy to see or feel and can manifest by redness, warmth, swelling, or pain around tissues or joints after an injury, like cutting yourself or falling. The immune system modulates its response to prevent further damage and facilitates healing and recovery. Examples of acute inflammation are flu, the common cold, bronchitis, headache, hives, or joint pain.

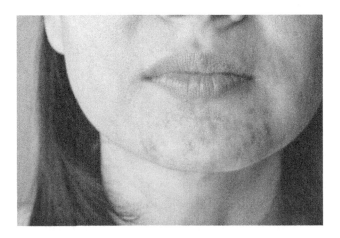

However, sometimes inflammation becomes self-perpetuating and lasts for months or even years, which is known as chronic inflammation. This serious condition can affect any part of the human body. It can also cause significant alterations in all tissues and organs. Recent evidence points to chronic inflammation as the most essential factor in promoting the formation and growth of plaque in arteries. Some studies have shown that the impact of chronic inflammation spans into growing areas of chronic disease.

Symptoms of Chronic Inflammation

Some of the common symptoms of chronic inflammation include:

- Body pain, arthralgia, myalgia
- Low Back Pain
- Skin symptoms, especially rashes
- Chronic fatigue, low energy, and insomnia
- Swollen Lymph Nodes
- Insulin Resistance
- Blood Clotting Problems
- Gastrointestinal complications like bloating and gas, abdominal pain, constipation, and diarrhea
- Excess Mucus Production
- Weight gain or weight loss
- Dry Eyes
- Frequent infections
- Depression, anxiety, brain fog, and mood disorders

Vitamin D and Chronic Inflammation

Much scientific and clinical literature currently exists on vitamin D and pregnancy due to the increasing awareness of the association between vitamin D adequacy and maternal and infant health outcomes. PUBMED (The National Library of Medicine, and the first source for biomedical literature) lists ≥ 5,698 publications that use the keywords "**vitamin D**" and "**inflammatory**" in either the title or abstract from 1947 to the present, with most of the research published in the last decade. This total includes publications that combine the use of the term "vitamin D" with one of the following terms:

- immune system (≥ 5,132 publications),
- immune response (≥ 3,140 publications),
- inflammation treatment (≥ 2,636 publications),
- psoriasis (≥ 1,748 publications),
- inflammation deficiency (≥ 1,720 publications)
- multiple sclerosis (≥ 1,642 publications),
- immunity (≥ 1,218 publications)
- rheumatoid arthritis (≥ 853 publications)

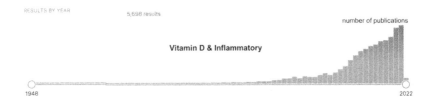

figure 3.1.1: increase in the number of articles published each year with the terms "inflammatory disease" and "vitamin D" in the title or abstract (in PUBMED.)

Besides being essential in calcium and phosphorus hemostasis, and bone health, vitamin D also exerts necessary functions for a healthy immune system. Vitamin D influences the immune cells to produce adapted and targeted actions against infections and avoid attacking the body's healthy cells.

Recent epidemiological studies have shown that vitamin D modulates the immune system to prevent tissue damage resulting from an excessive response. Low vitamin D status increases the risk of developing autoimmune diseases and infections.

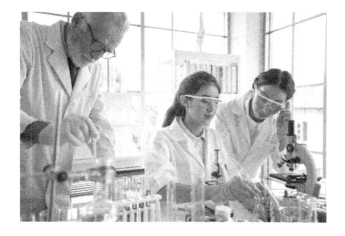

Evidence strongly links vitamin insufficiency with prevalent chronic autoimmune disorders such as multiple sclerosis, type 1 diabetes, Crohn's disease, and rheumatoid arthritis.

Recent studies shed light on the mechanisms that facilitate the role of vitamin D in modulating immune responses:

- regulation of the formation of inflammatory cytokines
- inhibition of the proliferation of pro-inflammatory cells

The clinical role of vitamin D in treating chronic inflammation and autoimmune disorders is auspicious, provided patients get adequate supplementation. Optimal vitamin D status is linked to a reduced risk of inflammation diseases for healthy people and positive outcomes in handling chronic inflammatory conditions for patients.

Chronic Inflammatory diseases

Inflammatory diseases are defined as persistent, chronic inflammations of one or more organs. Inflammatory conditions can affect most parts and organs of the human body: the nervous system, cardiovascular system, digestive system, epidermis, and joints.

Multiple Sclerosis (MS)

Multiple Sclerosis (MS) is a neuroinflammatory and neurodegenerative disorder characterized by neurological deficits ranging from mild to severe. MS is the most common disabling and devastating neurological disease in young adults between 20 to 40 years.

Multiple sclerosis occurs when the immune system mistakenly sends white blood cells to attack myelin coating —the insulation around nerve cells in the brain, optic nerves, and spinal cord. The immune system cells secrete chemicals that cause inflammation and destroy part of the myelin around some nerves, altering electrical messages in the brain. Patients with MS experience periods when symptoms get worse, known as relapses, and when symptoms get better, known as remission.

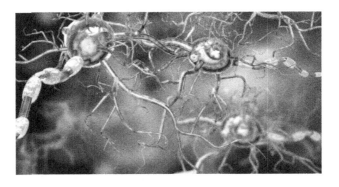

There are four main types of MS, classified as follows: relapsing-remitting MS (RRMS), secondary progressive MS (SPMS), primary progressive MS (PPMS), progressive relapsing MS (PRMS), and Benign Multiple Sclerosis (BMS).

Relapsing-remitting MS (RRMS): RRMS, the most common form of multiple sclerosis (80% of cases), affects women more often than men. RRMS is characterized by clearly defined attacks that symptoms come and go. Sudden symptoms or relapses follow periods of remission (absence of symptoms). The attacks can last from days to months.

Secondary progressive MS (SPMS): SPMS is a stage of multiple sclerosis that follows an initial relapsing-remitting MS for many patients. With this type of MS, symptoms progressively worsen over time because nerves are more damaged or lost at this stage. Patients with SPMS have fewer relapses than with RRMS due to decreased inflammation.

Progressive relapsing MS (PRMS): is the least common form, characterized by continual and progressive development and worsening from the beginning of symptoms over time.

Benign Multiple Sclerosis (BMS): BMS is a form of multiple sclerosis characterized by very mild attacks that do not worsen over time and show a good recovery.

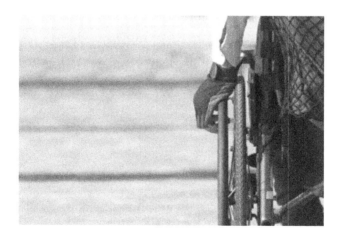

Many observational and epidemiological studies have been conducted to answer essential questions regarding vitamin D's impact on multiple sclerosis development and incidence.

A growing body of studies has shown that maintaining adequate levels of vitamin D (higher than 30 nanograms/mL (75 nmol/L) and in recent studies in the range of 40-60 nanograms/mL (100-150 nmol/L)) produce positive outcomes by reducing the risk of developing MS significantly.

Several epidemiological studies have shown that people living at higher latitudes are more likely to develop MS than those who live at lower latitudes or near the equator due to the lower exposure to ultraviolet B light. Additional studies focused on the link between vitamin D status and the risk of MS. They established that vitamin D insufficiency (< 30 nanograms/mL (<75 nmol/L)) is linked to a higher risk of developing MS both in women and men.

Recent studies have established that adequate vitamin D supplementation may have a therapeutic effect in treating multiple sclerosis. Optimal doses of vitamin D may effectively alter the course of multiple sclerosis. Thus an optimal vitamin D supplementation will decrease the risk of MS for healthy people and help reduce the frequency, symptoms, and severity of relapse episodes for patients with multiple sclerosis.

An optimal blood level of circulating vitamin D [25(OH)D] in the range of 40 and 60 nanograms/mL (100 and 150 nmol/L) will be associated with positive effects on MS.

Rheumatoid arthritis

Rheumatoid arthritis (RA) is an autoimmune and chronic inflammatory disorder that mainly affects joints, usually many joints at once. RA causes joint inflammation and pain. It occurs when the immune system starts to attack the lining of the joints by mistake. The disorder commonly affects joints in the hands, wrists, feet, spine, jaw, and knees. In joints, RA causes inflammation that induces pain, swelling, and stiffness. The RA disorder can also affect other body parts, such as the eyes, lungs, and heart.

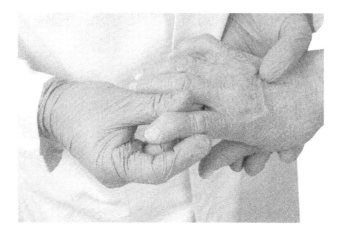

Although no cure exists for RA, early diagnosis and treatment can relieve symptoms, reduce the risk of joint deformity and lower the severity of the condition.

RA can be effectively treated with disease-modifying antirheumatic drugs (DMARDs) that slow disease and prevent joint damage. Surgery may sometimes be necessary to correct any joint problems that develop.

Rheumatoid arthritis (RA) has many functional and social consequences that influence the quality of life. RA **can vary widely in symptoms and outcomes.**

Having rheumatoid arthritis can lead to several adverse outcomes that can sometimes be life-threatening. RA can lead to:

- carpal tunnel syndrome is induced by the compression of the nerve controlling movement and sensation in the hands
- increased risk of heart attack
- increased risk of stroke
- inflammation of the lungs

- inflammation of the heart
- inflammation of eyes

Symptoms

Symptoms of rheumatoid arthritis may vary depending on many factors. They include:

- joint pain or aching
- joint stiffness worsens in the morning or usually after a period of inactivity.
- swelling, warmth, and redness in affected joints
- fatigue, tiredness, and a lack of energy
- loss of appetite
- weight loss
- chest pain—if the heart or lungs are affected
- Dry eyes and mouth—if the eyes are affected

Vitamin D for the management of rheumatoid arthritis

Vitamin D levels have been extensively studied in RA to investigate the existing associations and the potential role of vitamin D in treating RA.

Many observational and epidemiological studies have shown that low Vitamin D status is linked to increased susceptibility to the development of RA. Vitamin D insufficiency was found to be highly prevalent in patients with RA. Circulating vitamin D [25(OH)D] was inversely linked to RA condition severity. Thus patients with low vitamin D status are at greater risk of experiencing worsening symptoms and poor health outcomes. In addition, vitamin D deficiency is linked to the risk of other severe diseases, heart attack, stroke, inflammation of the lungs, inflammation of the heart, inflammation of the eyes, and osteoporosis. Thus, vitamin D is highly recommended for patients with RA to prevent these severe complications and relieve pain. Patients with RA have to correct their vitamin D status by achieving a vitamin D [25(OH)D] in the range of 40-60 nanograms/mL (100-150 nmol/L).

Psoriatic Arthritis

Psoriatic arthritis is a long-term immune-mediated condition involving inflammatory damage to certain joints or tendons. The affected joints become swollen, stiff, and painful. Over time, psoriatic arthritis can get severe, increasing the risk of the affected joints becoming damaged or deformed.

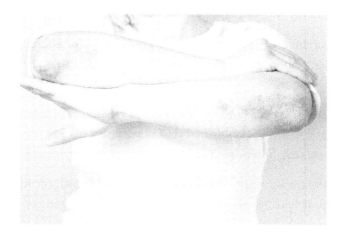

Although there currently is no cure for psoriatic arthritis, early diagnosis and treatments can slow its progress, lower its incidence, reduce pain, and protect the joints.

Symptoms of psoriatic arthritis

Psoriatic arthritis most often affects the large joints of the lower extremities, the fingers and toes, the back, and the pelvis. The symptoms of psoriatic arthritis may include:

- inflammation of all joints and phalanges of the fingers and toes,
- eye inflammation,
- fingers pain,
- wrists pain,
- knees pain,
- toes or ankles pain,
- nail changes, such as tiny bumps or crumbling,
- fatigue,
- anemia and moodiness,
- inflammatory bowel disease

Vitamin D for the management of Psoriatic Arthritis

The prevalence of low vitamin D status—(< 30 nanograms/mL (75 nmol/L))—among patients with psoriatic arthritis was around 82%, according to new studies.

Leading studies that examined the effect of vitamin D supplementation on psoriatic arthritis established that adequate amounts of vitamin D supplements might reduce symptoms in people with psoriatic arthritis.

The National Psoriasis Foundation Medical Board recommended that patients with psoriasis and/or psoriatic arthritis can get a vitamin D supplementation to their standard medical therapies to reduce disease severity.

In addition, several studies have shown that patients with psoriatic arthritis have an increased risk of osteoporosis due to coexisting conditions (for more details, please refer to chapter 2, "Osteoporosis and Vitamin D", Part III). Thus an optimal vitamin D supplementation will reduce the symptoms of psoriatic arthritis and decrease the risk of developing osteoporosis.

An optimal blood level of circulating vitamin D [25(OH)D] in the range of 40 and 60 nanograms/mL (100 and 150 nmol/L) may prevent breast cancer, improve the efficacy of chemotherapy and improve long-term survival for breast cancer patients

---

Systemic lupus erythematosus (lupus)

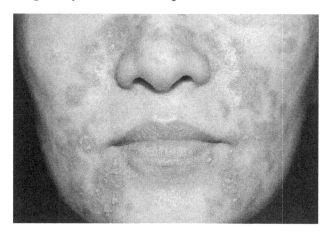

Systemic lupus erythematosus—often called "lupus"— is a chronic disease that can affect people of all ages, with a high predominance of women (90% of new patients). Lupus is a multisystem autoimmune inflammatory condition that can affect all organs and parts of the body with varying clinical manifestations in patients.

Lupus happens when the immune system mistakenly attacks connective tissues throughout the body (skin, brain, heart, joints, lungs, liver, kidneys). It varies from mild mucocutaneous manifestations to severe life-threatening conditions involving vital organs.

Although no cure exists for lupus, some treatments may help improve symptoms, prevent flares, and prevent health complications caused by lupus.

Diagnosis of lupus may be challenging because most of the symptoms are common with other diseases. Patients may have lupus for a while without knowing it, which makes early diagnosis difficult.

Effective treatments can help lower the damaging effects of lupus, reduce the severity of symptoms and lower the risk of complications caused by lupus.

Symptoms

People with lupus experience periods of disease symptoms, called flares, with variable frequencies and periods of absence of symptoms, called remission. Symptoms include:

- prolonged or extreme fatigue
- fever
- skin rashes,
- pain or swelling in the joints
- muscle pain
- chest pain
- headaches
- hair loss
- anemia
- memory problems
- blood clotting problems
- dry eyes, eye inflammation
- mouth ulcers

Vitamin D for the management of Psoriatic Arthritis

Multiple studies have shown that most patients with lupus have insufficient levels of circulating vitamin D [25(OH)D]. Vitamin D insufficiency is associated with worsening symptoms, increased risk for permanent organ damage, and maybe more extended periods of flares. In addition, low vitamin D status is associated with increased disease activity and worsening symptoms such as joint pains, extreme and prolonged fatigue, and fever.

Patients with lupus experience abnormal activity in the skin of apoptosis —the cellular programmed death process by which the body kills the damaged cells—. This may lead to more inflammation, worsening of skin lesions, and more generalized and unusual skin reactions to light. This last condition is photosensitivity and poses a severe problem for lupus patients, deepening the vitamin D deficiency. Studies have confirmed that roughly 70% of patients with lupus have abnormal sensitivity to ultraviolet rays, either from sunlight or artificial sources. In addition, excess sun exposure causes frequent flares and triggers lupus symptoms.

Other studies examined the association between vitamin D insufficiency and the exacerbation of lupus symptoms. They confirmed that low vitamin D status is associated with morbidity and mortality in patients with lupus. As photosensitivity is a prevalent condition, patients are advised to avoid sunlight, which causes poorer vitamin D status. Thus, oral vitamin D supplementation is the unique viable alternative for patients to correct their vitamin D status.

Accumulating evidence confirms that patients with lupus who have low vitamin D status (<30 nanograms/mL) are at high risk of developing cardiovascular illnesses, metabolic syndrome, and insulin resistance. Thus, correcting vitamin D status and achieving an optimal vitamin D status in the range of **50 and 80 nanograms/mL (125 to 200 nmol/L)** —which corresponds to the preventive cancer range— is necessary to prevent other chronic diseases, improve long-term lupus-related outcomes for patients with lupus.

Please refer to the chapter "vitamin D optimal doses" in Part II for detailed information on achieving your desired vitamin D status.

19

INFECTIOUS DISEASES

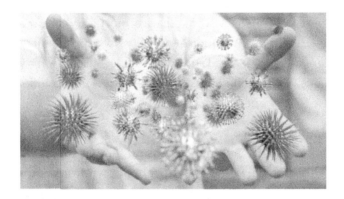

Optimal Vitamin D status is associated with reduced risk of being infected with COVID-19, decreased severity of COVID-19, and lower mortality from COVID-19, even for high-risk populations—older adults, pregnant women, people with underlying medical conditions like diabetes, cardiovascular and chronic respiratory disease, obesity and cancer.

Infectious diseases are a leading cause of mortality and morbidity in all parts of the world and constitute a major public health concern. Infectious diseases are illnesses caused by various microorganisms—typically viruses, bacteria, fungi, worms, parasites, and protozoans—that enter the body, multiply, cause an infection, and impair the person's health. Several infectious disorders are contagious and spread from one person to another. They can sometimes be caught from the environment, insect bites, or animal contact.

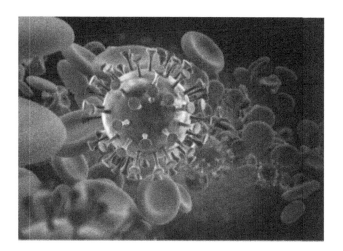

Usually, when the person's immune system works as expected—with appropriate responses— disease symptoms may not develop. In contrast, autoimmune symptoms may develop if the host immune system over-reacts and produces an abnormal immune response. The infectious disease develops if the patient's immune system is weak/compromised or the infectious microorganism overwhelms the immune system.

With the development of antibiotics therapies and immunization protocols, it seemed that infectious diseases, particularly bacterial infections, would no longer constitute a significant public health problem. However, with the emergence of drug-resistant bacteria and deadly viral diseases such as severe acute respiratory syndrome (COVID-19), the world is struggling with rising deadly infections.

Infectious diseases may be divided as:

- foodborne and waterborne infections refer to illnesses caused by consuming foods or beverages infected by various bacteria, viruses, and parasites.
- waterborne infections refer to illnesses caused by ingesting water contaminated by viruses, parasites, and bacteria.
- deadly illnesses like COVID-19, Ebola and anthrax
- diseases spread by vectors —mosquitoes, ticks, and fleas
- disorders caused by contact with animals
- conditions that are resistant to antibiotics

Some Common Infectious illnesses:

- Severe acute respiratory syndrome (SARS)
- Sexually transmitted diseases
- Common cold
- Influenza (flu)
- Pertussis (whooping cough)
- Diphtheria
- Escherichia coli
- HIV/AIDS
- Lyme disease
- Malaria
- Meningitis
- Pneumonia
- Salmonella infections
- Shingles (herpes zoster)
- Tuberculosis
- Viral hepatitis

Signs and symptoms

The signs and symptoms of an infectious disease are specific and sometimes uncommon, like hemorrhagic fever. General typical signs and symptoms include:

- fever
- diarrhea
- loss of appetite
- fatigue
- muscles aches and pains
- coughing

Vitamin D and Infectious Diseases

Much scientific and clinical literature currently exists on vitamin D and pregnancy due to the increasing awareness of the association between vitamin D adequacy and maternal and infant health outcomes. PUBMED (The National Library of Medicine, and the first source for biomedical literature) lists ≥ 6,311 publications that use the keywords "**vitamin D**" and "**infection**" in either the title or abstract from 1945 to the present, with most of the research published in the last decade. This total includes publications that combine the use of the term "vitamin D" with one of the following terms:

- infection treatment (≥ 3,683 publications),
- infection deficiency (vitamin D) (≥ 2,618 publications),
- infection prevention (≥ 1,448 publications),
- tuberculosis (≥ 1,209 publications),
- COVID-19 (≥ 1,002 publications),
- pneumonia (≥ 991 publications),
- HIV/AIDS (≥ 790 publications),
- influenza (≥ 250 publications),
- escherichia coli (≥ 183 publications)

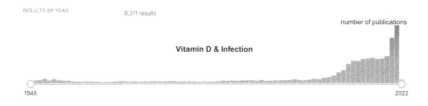

RESULTS BY YEAR   6,311 results

number of publications

Vitamin D & Infection

1945   2022

figure 3.1.1: increase in the number of articles published each year with the terms "infection" and "vitamin D" in the title or abstract (in PUBMED.)

COVID-19

COVID-19—identified in Wuhan, China—is a highly contagious infectious respiratory illness caused by the SARS-CoV-2 virus. The new coronavirus was discovered in 2019 in China and mainly spread from person to person through droplets produced when an infected person sneezes, coughs, or talks.

Symptoms of COVID-19

The symptoms of this illness are diverse due to the capacity of the virus to affect any organ in the body of a COVID-19 patient.

Most people who are infected may never develop signs or have minor symptoms. However, the disease can vary from mild to severe for people with symptoms.

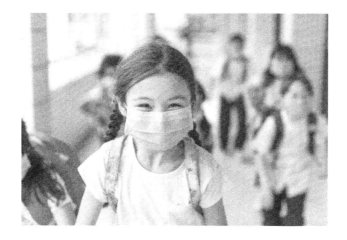

Mild to moderate symptoms (81%) include:

- fever or chills. Fever appears to be one of the more common early symptoms of COVID-19. Fever may be accompanied or not by Chills.
- continuous cough. Most COVID-19 patients have a dry and continuous cough they can feel in their chest. COVID-19 may invade the lungs, irritate the respiratory tract and cause persistent dry cough.
- new loss of taste or smell. Smell and taste dysfunctions are common among COVID-19-infected people. Nearly half of COVID-19 patients experience a suddenly lost sense of smell and/or taste.

Other symptoms include:

- fatigue,
- congestion or runny nose,
- shortness of breath or difficulty breathing
- mild pneumonia,
- muscle or body aches
- headache
- sore throat

- nausea or vomiting
- diarrhea

People over 65 years and those of any age with underlying medical conditions like diabetes, cardiovascular disease, chronic respiratory disease, obesity, and cancer are at higher risk of developing severe illnesses. Patients who develop severe COVID-19 may experience some or all the common COVID-19 symptoms and signs described above, along with:

- severe shortness of breath
- chest discomfort, persistent pain or pressure in the chest
- inability to wake or stay awake
- grey, or blue-colored skin, face, nail beds, or lips (a sign patient not getting enough oxygen)
- confusion and unresponsiveness

Complications and Sequelae

The COVID-19 virus attacks the respiratory tract and other vital and non-vital organs in the human body. This lead to various complication and sequelae for patients who have severe illnesses:

- respiratory system complications include respiratory failure, acute respiratory distress syndrome, pulmonary fibrosis, and chronic lung disease.
- cardiovascular system complications include cardiomyopathy, arrhythmias, acute coronary syndrome, conduction system malfunction, myocardial injury, heart attacks, and heart failure.
- nervous system complications include stroke, muscle and nerve damage, cerebrovascular disorders, encephalitis, and impairment of consciousness.
- endocrine system complications include insulin resistance in

people with type 2 diabetes, pancreas injury, thyroid dysfunction, and impaired spermatogenesis in men.

Vitamin D and COVID-19

Vitamin D has direct antiviral effects primarily against enveloped viruses, and coronavirus is an enveloped virus.

Several studies established a strong association between circulating vitamin D [25OHD] and the outcomes of COVID-19 infection, particularly the risk of developing symptoms, severity, and mortality. Low vitamin D status is linked with an increased risk of COVID-19 infection and for the high-risk population with bad outcomes.

Many studies have established the efficacy of vitamin D supplementation, magnesium, and zinc in preventing or treating COVID-19. The optimal doses of vitamin D, with the protocol to improve your vitamin D status, are presented in the chapter "vitamin D optimal doses". This will allow you to get the full benefits of vitamin D, prevent COVID-19 infection, lower its severity, and significantly reduce the risk of complications.

Maintaining an adequate vitamin D status between 50 and 70 nanograms/mL (125 to 175 nmol/L) for both women and men will significantly reduce the risk of being infected by the COVID-19 virus or experiencing severe illness.

Please refer to the chapter "vitamin D optimal doses" in Part II for detailed information on achieving your desired vitamin D status.

20

OSTEOPOROSIS AND VITAMIN D

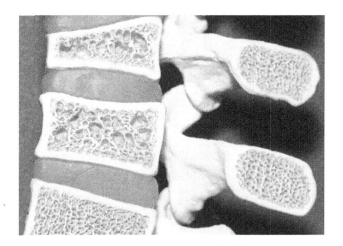

Vitamin D promotes calcium and phosphorus absorption from the intestines, followed by reabsorption by the kidneys. Indispensable for growth during infancy, it ensures the strength of the human skeleton and prevents osteoporosis. Low vitamin D status is associated with an increased risk of bone disorders and altered health.

Osteoporosis is a degenerative disorder characterized by a gradual loss of bone mass that affects 200 million people around the world. In the United States, around 10 million adults—80 percent of women—have hip osteoporosis. An additional 33.6 million people over age 50 suffer from osteopenia —low bone mass— of the hip and thus are at high risk of developing osteoporosis.

Osteoporosis signifies "porous bone." If you observe healthy bones under a microscope, they look like a honeycomb (see figure 3.6.1). When osteoporosis develops, the bone tissue structure changes, and the spaces and holes in the honeycomb become much larger than in healthy bone due to the loss of density or mass.

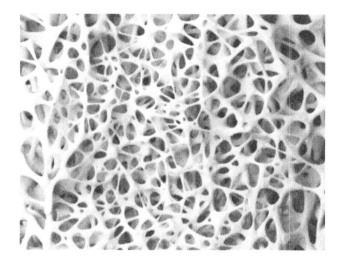

figure 3.6.1

Since osteoporosis is a condition in which some bones become less dense and more likely to fracture, its diagnosis measures bone density and evaluates fracture risk. Thus, your doctor will most likely order a Bone DXA (dual-energy x-ray absorptiometry) to measure your bone mineral density (BMD). In most cases, only the hip and lumbar spine are checked.

The DXA machine uses low X-rays, measures the amounts of x-rays absorbed by bone and tissues, and correlates with bone mineral density.

Diagnosis Of Osteoporosis

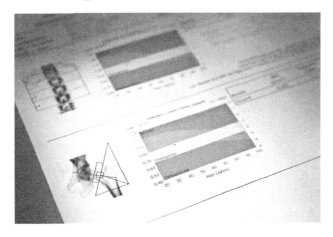

Since osteoporosis is a condition in which some bones become less dense and more likely to fracture, its diagnosis measures bone density and evaluates fracture risk. Thus, your doctor will most likely order a Bone DXA (dual-energy x-ray absorptiometry) to measure your bone mineral density (BMD). In most cases, only the hip and lumbar spine are checked.

The DXA machine uses low X-rays, measures the amounts of x-rays absorbed by bone and tissues, and correlates with bone mineral density.

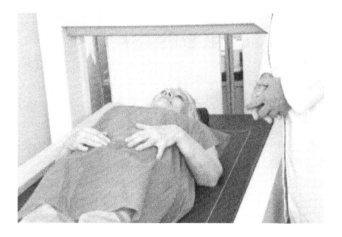

The DXA machine performs some conversions to estimate your bone density information through your T and Z scores. T-score is measured by comparing your bone density to the average population of young adults and is used to determine your risk of developing a fracture and the need for drug therapy. Your Z score is measured by comparing your bone density to those in your age group. This score can indicate if further medical tests are needed.

Risk Factors for Osteoporosis

Many conditions or factors increase your risk for osteoporosis. They include:

- **vitamin D deficiency.** Low vitamin D levels may raise your risk of developing osteoporosis and broken bones.
- **advancing age.** The process of bone growth (bone remodeling) slows down as someone ages, inducing a higher risk for osteoporotic fractures.
- **sex.** women are at a greater risk than men due to naturally lower bone mass and thinner bones.
- **genetic background.** A family history of the disease is identified as a risk factor for developing osteoporosis and bone fracture.
- **diabetes type I.** It is established that patients with type I

diabetes are six times more likely to experience osteoporosis and bone fractures due to low bone mass. In patients with type 2 diabetes, the risk is increased by twice due to the low quality of bone.

- **history of fractures.** A history of broken bones or fragility fractures at an age higher than 45 may indicate an increased risk of osteoporosis.
- **menopause.** Lower estrogen levels at menopause impact the bone remodeling process and accelerate bone loss, causing decreased bone strength and higher fracture risk.
- **menstrual history in women.** Abnormal absence of menstrual periods or light menstruation throughout life may lead to a higher risk for osteoporosis.
- **low testosterone in males.** Low testosterone levels in men may influence bone growth and induce osteoporosis.
- **cigarette smoking.** Several observational studies have identified smoking as a risk factor for bone fracture and osteoporosis.
- **alcohol consumption.** Several observational studies have established that chronic alcohol consumption can trigger.
- **irregular menstrual cycles.** It is established that the irregular menstrual cycle constitutes a risk factor for osteoporosis and bone fracture.
- **physical inactivity.** A sedentary lifestyle characterized by little physical exercise is associated with bone mass loss and an increased risk of osteoporosis and bone fracture.
- **chronic use of some drugs.** Prolonged consumption of
- certain medications, like those used to treat asthma, thyroid, and lupus deficiencies, are associated with an increased risk of osteoporosis.
- **vitamin K2 deficiency.** Observational studies have identified that poor Vitamin K intake is associated with bone mass loss, osteoporosis, and fracture risk.

Vitamin D and Bone Disease

Numerous scientific and clinical literature currently exists on vitamin D and osteoporosis due to the classical association between vitamin D adequacy and bone health. PUBMED (The National Library of Medicine, and the first source for biomedical literature) lists ≥ 10,760 publications that use the keywords "**vitamin D**" and "**osteoporosis**" in either the title or abstract from 1935 to the present, with most of the research published in the last three decades. This total includes publications that combine the use of vitamin D with one of the following terms:

- osteoporosis treatment (≥ 7,808 publications)
- osteoporosis prevention (≥ 4,582 publications),
- osteoporosis older adults (≥ 5,523 publications),
- osteoporosis women (≥ 3,797 publications),
- osteoporosis deficiency (≥ 2,978 publications),
- osteoporosis status (≥ 1,585 publications).

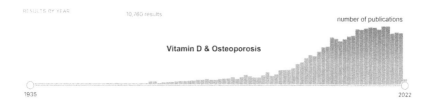

figure 3.1.1: increase in the number of articles published each year with the terms "osteoporosis" and "vitamin D" in the title or abstract (in PUBMED.)

Treatment of osteoporosis

The primary treatment combines vitamin D and calcium supplements with adequate medication and an adapted exercise program. If osteoporosis results from prolonged use of a drug (corticosteroid therapy, etc.), drug use is quickly stopped.

Several drugs, including Cisphosphonates, Calcitonin can slow down bone degeneration while significantly reducing the risk of fractures. In addition, it is often possible to regain some of the lost bone mass.

Vitamin D deficiency and osteoporosis

Vitamin D is essential for the normal development and maintenance of your skeleton. Vitamin D deficiency was first associated with rickets in children and osteomalacia in adults. Many studies have established the hormonally active vitamin D form [1,25(OH)2D] promotes calcium absorption from the gut, and poor vitamin D status leads to not having enough vitamin D to be converted in the [1,25(OH)2D] form. Thus, vitamin D deficiency leads to osteoporosis, fractures, mineralization defects, and muscle weakness.

Recent studies have also established that vitamin D adequacy is associated with optimal bone mineral density and bone remodeling. Vitamin D supplementation was shown to be essential in increasing bone mineral density. Supplementing with vitamin D alone or in combination with calcium was associated with reducing the incidence of hip, vertebral, and other non-vertebral fractures in older adults.

Vitamin D supplementation and osteoporosis

Maintaining an adequate vitamin D status between 40 and 60 nanograms/mL (100 to 150 nmol/L) for both women and men will prevent osteoporosis and other bone disorders.

If you already have osteoporosis, you should reach and maintain optimal vitamin D [25(OH)D] levels equal to or greater than 60 nanograms/mL (150 nmol/L).

Please refer to the chapter "vitamin D optimal doses" in Part II for detailed information on how to achieve your desired vitamin D status.

21

SELECTED QUESTIONS & ANSWERS ON VITAMIN D

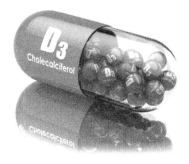

What is vitamin D, and why does the human body need it?

Vitamin D is a hormone our bodies make and a nutrient we eat. Vitamin D2 and D3 are produced when solar-ultraviolet B radiation interacts with a form of cholesterol. The making of vitamin D by the human body is triggered when solar-ultraviolet B (UVB) hits the skin and constitutes the main vitamin D body's supply. Vitamin D plays a crucial role by enabling the body to absorb and retain calcium and phosphorus and promotes bone health. Vitamin D promotes bone health and overall health and prevents many diseases, including cancers, type 2 diabetes, cardiovascular diseases, autoimmunity disease, kidney and liver disease, bone disorders, depression, anxiety, and infections.

How much vitamin D do I need?

The reference value for vitamin D intake is from the government's recommendations. Recommended dietary allowances (RDAs) for vitamin D are listed in the table below in both micrograms (mcg or μg) and international units (IU).

Age	Male	Female	Pregnancy	Lactation
0-12 months	10 mcg (400 IU)	10 mcg (400 IU)		
1–13 years	15 mcg (600 IU)	15 mcg (600 IU)		
14–18 years	15 mcg (600 IU)	15 mcg (600 IU)	15 mcg (600 IU)	15 mcg (600 IU)
19–50 years	15 mcg (600 IU)	15 mcg (600 IU)	15 mcg (600 IU)	15 mcg (600 IU)
51–70 years	15 mcg (600 IU)	15 mcg (600 IU)		
>70 years	20 mcg (800 IU)	20 mcg (800 IU)		

These values correspond to the amount of vitamin D that will prevent rickets and osteomalacia in healthy people. Much higher amounts are needed for individuals with an increased risk of vitamin D deficiency.

In Part II, you'll learn more about optimal doses of vitamin D intake.

What are the upper limits of vitamin D intake?

Tolerable Upper Intake Levels (ULs) are the maximum daily intakes that are safe (unlikely to cause adverse health effects.)

In this last decade, experts have reevaluated the safety of using vitamin D and provided revised reference values. For adults, two European studies have suggested that a 250 μg vitamin D daily intake

(10.000 IU) is considered safe with no observed adverse effect level. Despite this body of evidence, the panels of experts established the UL for all adults, including lactating and pregnant women, to 100 µg/day (4.000 IU/day). The UL was set to 100 µg/day (4.000 IU/day) for ages 11-17. For children aged 1-10 years, the UL was adapted to 50 µg/day (2.000 IU/day), considering their smaller body size. The UL was set to 25 µg/day for infants under one year (1.000 IU/day).

How can the vitamin D supply be defined?

Suppose the reference value for vitamin D intake is 15 mcg per day. If a person lives above the 37-degree latitude line —roughly the imaginary line between Philadelphia and San Francisco— in the northern hemisphere, the body's own (endogenous) production in the skin is near zero in the autumn and winter months. He needs to get his 15 mcg of vitamin D per day through customary foods (5 to 15 percent) and 85 to 95 percent through dietary supplementation.

In summer, the body's endogenous production in the skin may account for 80 to 90 percent of vitamin D supply.

To calculate the time you need in the sun to get your dose of vitamin D3 without the risk of sunburn, you are advised to use this online calculator developed by Ola Engelsen, a scientist in the Department of Atmosphere and Climate at the Norwegian Institute for Air Research.

The calculator is available at this address:

(https://fastrt.nilu.no/VitD_quartMEDandMED_v2.html)

What is the vitamin D status of the American Population? Is there a supply gap?

The vitamin D status of the U.S. population has been monitored since 1988 by the National Health and Nutrition Examination Survey (NHANES). The monitoring measures blood 25(OH)D levels according to many factors, including age, gender, racial group, vitamin D supplement users, and non-users...

The entire group that took a vitamin D supplement increased from 23 percent in 1988—1994 to 35 percent in 2009—2010.

Although some progress has been made during this timeframe, vitamin D levels overall in the U.S. population remain low. That means that a large percentage of the population is suffering from vitamin D deficiency or insufficiency or not benefiting from the preventive potential of vitamin D for bone health and overall health.

How much sun exposure does the body need to produce an adequate vitamin D amount by itself? How does winter compare to summer?

The body's vitamin D production in the skin depends on several factors, including residence latitude, season, time of the day, clothing, weather conditions clothing, time spent outdoors, age, weight status, skin type, and the use of sun-blocking products. That means that the body's vitamin D production may differ enormously from one individual to another. So for an accurate calculation of your body's production, you are advised to use this online calculator developed by Ola Engelsen, a scientist in the Department of Atmosphere and Climate at the Norwegian Institute for Air Research.

The calculator is available at this address:

(https://fastrt.nilu.no/VitD_quartMEDandMED_v2.html)

Thanks to vitamin D cutaneous photosynthesis, you can reach the desired serum concentration of 25(OH)D of 50 nmol/L in the summer months. Again, you are advised to use the online calculator to appreciate the influence of the season on your body's production.

Thus you'll find that adults (skin types 1,2, and 3) —with 25 percent of body exposure to the sun every day between 12 noon and 3 pm for 5 to 30 minutes— will produce all their vitamin D needs.

However, except in the summer, people living above the 35th parallel latitude from October to March will not meet their vitamin D requirements. The body's vitamin D production is near zero in the winter months.

How does the body store vitamin D?

Like other fat-soluble vitamins, the excess vitamin D is stored in the body's adipose tissue (fat) for later use. That means your body can mobilize its reserves when needed. This storage mechanism extends the vitamin D total-body half-life to approximately two months in the body.

Should I take a vitamin D supplement?

People in the northern parts of the U.S. above the 37-degree latitude line —roughly the imaginary line between Philadelphia and San Francisco— get little to no UVB exposure between the autumn and winter months to make vitamin D. So you'll require supplements to get the vitamin D you need. Consider also the foods you eat; you can get 5-15 percent of your need.

1

REFERENCES

PubMed database (National Library of Medicine) was used primarily for the selection of many articles used throughout this book.

https://pubmed.ncbi.nlm.nih.gov/

ABOUT THE AUTHOR

"Dr. H. Maher" is a joint pen name under which Dr. Y. Naitlho, PharmD, and H. Naitlho, MS/MBA, co-write books.

Dr. Y. Naitlho PharmD has over 25 years of pharmacy practice, applied nutrition research, and writing. He is currently a pharmacist and health and nutrition writer. He is the author of several books in the field of food science and human nutrition, and applied nutrition.

Dr. Y. Naitlho received his Doctor of Pharmacy from Perm State Pharmaceutical Academy. As a pharmacist and nutrition professional, He ensures that book design meets readers' dynamic learning needs and that content meets reliability and integrity standards.

H. Naitlho has over 30 years of engineering practice and science and engineering Research. He is the author of several books in the field of business management and coauthor of numerous books in food science and human nutrition, food engineering, and applied nutrition.

H. Naitlho holds an Engineering degree from the École Supérieure d'Aéronautique et de l'Espace (Sup'Aéro), an Engineering degree from the École de l'Air (Salon de Provence) and has an MBA from Laureate International Universities, a post-graduate degree in Automatics from Paul Sabatier University, and a further post-graduate degree in Mechanics from Aix Marseille University.

H. Naitlho brings the engineering mindset and scientific rigor. He consistently refines ideas, analyzes data, and carries consistency and a great sense of detail to their work.